f

Diagnosing Genius

DIAGNOSING GENIUS

The Life and Death
of Beethoven

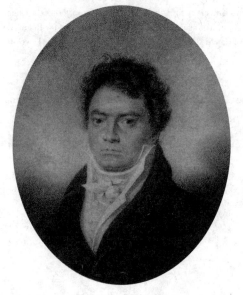

FRANÇOIS MARTIN MAI

McGill-Queen's University Press
Montreal & Kingston · London · Ithaca

© McGill-Queen's University Press 2007
ISBN 978-0-7735-3190-1

Legal deposit first quarter 2007
Bibliothèque nationale du Québec

Printed in Canada on acid-free paper

This book has been published with the help of a grant from the Guthrie Trust.

McGill-Queen's University Press acknowledges the support of the Canada Council for the Arts for our publishing program. We also acknowledge the financial support of the Government of Canada through the Book Publishing Industry Development Program (BPIDP) for our publishing activities.

LIBRARY AND ARCHIVES CANADA CATALOGUING IN PUBLICATION

Mai, François Martin
Diagnosing genius : the life and death of Beethoven / François Martin Mai.
Includes bibliographical references and index.
ISBN 978-0-7735-3190-1
1. Beethoven, Ludwig van, 1770–1827 – Health.
2. Genius and mental illness   I. Title.
ML410.B4M217 2007   780'.92   C2006-905669-2

Set in 11/15 Bulmer Std
Book design & typesetting by Garet Markvoort, zijn digital

This book is dedicated to the memory of my parents
Martin Mai and Yvonne Nadaud
who stimulated my interest in medicine,
in music, and in history.

CONTENTS

FOREWORD

Beethoven is such an icon for music lovers that one is almost compelled to picture him as superhuman. Yes, we all know that he became severely deaf, but his ability to transcend this handicap and continue his artistic triumphs only adds to the mystique enveloping him. He is the hero who could revolutionize music, fraternize on the basis of equality with the intelligentsia, the nobility, and the aristocracy, hold discourses on philosophy, politics, music, and art in general, and prevail over human frailty to create immortal masterpieces. He has stirred so many of us so profoundly that we feel a love and an affinity for him that transcends the rational. Thus in some ways it may be even more unpleasant and painful to read about Beethoven's bouts of diarrhea, his depressions, the litres of fluid drained from his body, and the primitive medical modalities applied to him than to hear about the suffering of our own friends and relatives, who at least in some cases may be receiving appropriate and effective treatment for their maladies.

Is it then some sort of malignant curiosity that leads us to delve into the details of his morbidity and sift through reams of documentation on his afflictions? Is he not entitled to some posthumous privacy about his bodily functions and his demise? It seems that great geniuses, just like holders or seekers of public office, have no possibility of drawing a curtain over any aspect of their lives. In the case of the latter, the preservation of integrity and the prevention of corruption and abuse of power dictate transparency. As for the geniuses, those who have created the best that man is capable of, their confrontation with life is simply too central to our understanding of our own lives to allow anything to remain hidden.

It is not always a pretty picture – neither the bodily nor the moral failings. We would rather that Richard Strauss had not had lunch with Hitler, that Wagner had not been anti-Semitic, and that Balakirev had not been a member of the virulent "Black Hundreds," yet we do not hide these facts and must come to terms with them.

Aside from the compelling interest in the lives of genius, this book also provides a fascinating opportunity to watch and study the details of medical care two hundred years ago. The astounding amount of detail in this case history is available only because of Beethoven's great fame, even during his lifetime. No comparable medical portrait could be assembled for some anonymous burger of the day because no one would have had such a great interest in documenting and preserving all the facts. While almost everyone is aware that Beethoven was deaf, his many other ailments, both physical and mental, are not so well known. Professor Mai's book thoroughly documents the massive evidence of the composer's life-long struggle with a debilitating array of health problems.

Mai's final chapter discusses and illuminates the puzzling relationship between genius, creativity, and various degrees of mental abnormality. It seems that, at least in many cases, the suffering caused by the latter is almost a prerequisite for the second. Yet often the work created during the artist's most tormented periods does not reflect that agony but perhaps serves as a self-created attempt to escape to a happier universe of the imagination, which can then serve as therapy to help alleviate the artist's pain.

Professor Mai approaches his subject both as a scientist and as a medical detective, weighing possibilities and probabilities in a carefully reasoned manner. He does not impose definitive answers on all the open questions but he certainly presents us with all the evidence needed to speculate and create our own image of this extraordinary human being who has meant so much to so many, for such a long time.

Anton Kuerti
November 2006
http://www.jwentworth.com/kuerti

PREFACE

Beethoven is an iconic figure in human history. Many who know nothing about classical music have heard of Ludwig van Beethoven, know about his deafness, and are aware of his reputation as a composer. His music is widely played and heard, and, with the possible exception of Mozart, his compositions are the most appreciated by music lovers.

We are fortunate to know a great deal about his life. He was a copious letter writer, particularly during his middle and later years. We have more than 1,500 extant letters, written to family, friends, publishers, and others. Because of his contemporary fame, many of his friends and admirers wrote about him, both during his life and after his death, providing descriptions of his appearance and personality and anecdotes about events in his life. These documents represent a bountiful source of information for his biographers. But there also are many gaps in our knowledge, and this lack of information has stimulated debate and controversy about various aspects of his life, including his relationships and his health problems. Medical and non-medical experts have argued about the causes of his deafness and his final illness, and about whether or not he had syphilis or abused alcohol. As new information comes to light, our perspective can change. For example, Maynard Solomon deduced the identity of the long mysterious "Immortal Beloved" in the 1970s, and in the 1990s Alfredo Guevara, William Walsh, and their colleagues discovered that Beethoven's hair contained high quantities of lead.

There has been an abiding interest in Beethoven's health and illnesses since shortly after his death in 1827. Much has been written by physicians about this topic, but almost all of this literature is in professional medical journals, and access is not always easy for the general public. Many are intrigued by the question of how a person who lacks the sensory system that most regard as essential for musical composition – the ability to hear the results of one's creative efforts – can nevertheless compose serene and sublime music. What is not so widely known is that Beethoven suffered a number of health problems aside from his deafness, conditions that affected his gastrointestinal, respiratory, and musculoskeletal systems, his eyes, and, not least, his mental state. Judging from his letters, one can say that he had a lifelong preoccupation – some call it hypochondriacal – with health.

This book presents a discussion of Beethoven's life, health, death, and creativity. It begins with a description of the political, social, and medical climate in Europe during Beethoven's lifetime, and outlines how the revolutionary nature of Beethoven's music reflected the political and social upheavals and revolutions during this period. It also describes the state of medicine and health care in early nineteenth-century Europe, in order to provide a context for the diagnoses made by his physicians and the medical treatments to which he was subjected. Chapter 2 provides a brief biography of Beethoven with emphasis on his family, character, health, and relationships, particularly those with women. His music is mentioned only in the context of these aspects of his life. Although controversies continue as to how Beethoven's life and music should be categorized, this text follows the traditional division into four periods. Chapter 3 presents the factual details about Beethoven's health as he himself described his symptoms and his problems in letters and as these illnesses and events were reported by others, including his physicians. Primary source material presented in this context includes a new translation of the autopsy report from the original Latin as well as excerpts from the Conversation Books (writing pads that Beethoven used in order to enable others to communicate with him when their speech was no longer audible to him) that have not previously been available in English. Chapter 4 formulates and interprets this health information in the context of modern clinical medicine.

The final chapter reviews the psychology of creativity, and discusses the effects of medical and psychiatric illness on creativity in art, literature, and musical composition in an attempt to answer the question: How was it possible for Beethoven to compose such awe-inspiring music, in spite of the fact that he was experiencing many serious health problems for a major part of his life? The last few decades have seen a growing fascination with the creative process, and many questions have been posed about the nature and expression of eminent creativity. What factors are associated with creativity, and what factors promote or impair it? Biographical data indicate that many creative individuals have difficult lives and personalities. How does this affect their creativity? How are they able to overcome these difficulties and yet remain creative? This book explores, and attempts to answer some of these questions in relation to the life and the music of Ludwig van Beethoven.

ACKNOWLEDGMENTS

There are difficulties in bridging disciplines as different as medicine, music and history, and I would like to thank the many individuals who gave of their time and expertise to help me take on this challenge.

My medical colleagues, Drs John Henderson, André Lamothe, Andrew Mai, Egils Mierins, Jean Michaud, George Mintsioulis, John Seely, and Grant Thompson read pertinent extracts of the medical chapters and gave invaluable advice on their specialty areas.

Anne Weiser translated Dr Johann Schmidt's letter to Beethoven into English, and reviewed early drafts of the manuscript. Fr Frank Morrisey OMI translated Beethoven's autopsy report from the original Latin. Gaëtan Béllec, Noel Burns, Donna Burr, Bill Burr, David Currie, Marguerite Macdonald, and Jim Morrisey reviewed various drafts of the manuscript and made many useful factual and other recommendations. Special thanks are due to Gretchen Conrad and Laurel O'Connor who read the manuscript meticulously and made many helpful suggestions. Anton Kuerti reviewed the manuscript and made many valuable recommendations. I am particularly grateful that he also agreed to write the Foreword to this book. Despite this substantial input, any errors of fact or interpretation belong solely to the author.

I would like to express my appreciation to Bill Meredith and Patricia Stroh of the Ira F. Brilliant Center for Beethoven Studies of San Jose State

University, California; to Drs Sieghard Brandenburg and Nicole Kämp-ken of Beethoven-Haus, in Bonn, Germany; and to the Pathologische-Anatomisches Bundesmuseum in Vienna for their support and permission to use images and documents located in these centres. My thanks are also due to the Guthrie Trust of Edinburgh, Scotland for a financial grant, and to my son Quentin for assistance. My editors Joan Harcourt, Joan McGilvray, and Ruth Pincoe of McGill-Queen's University Press have provided great support and editorial direction.

Finally, this project could never have been begun or completed without the invaluable and unfailing help of my wife, Sarie, during the six years that the manuscript has been in gestation. We have had extended diurnal and nocturnal discussions about Beethoven, and her perspicacity has helped to generate many ideas that have helped my understanding of his health, his life, and his relationships.

Diagnosing Genius

CHAPTER ONE

The Setting

Mozart's genius still mourns and is weeping over the death of its pupil. In the inexhaustible Haydn, it found refuge but no occupation; through him it wishes to form union with another. Through uninterrupted diligence you shall receive Mozart's spirit from Haydn's hands.

> Written by Count Ferdinand Waldstein to Beethoven in October 1792 when the young musician left Bonn for Vienna.[1]

The year is 1804. Napoleon Bonaparte has decided to crown himself Emperor of France. Europe is in a period of brief and uneasy peace after fifteen years of political turmoil generated by the French Revolution. Like millions of other Europeans, Ludwig van Beethoven, aged thirty-three, had been strongly influenced by the ideals of the Revolution. He had developed an admiration for Napoleon, the First Consul of France, and believed that Napoleon would crystallize these ideals by creating a more liberal society. Beethoven conceived and wrote one of his greatest works, the Symphony no. 3, op. 55 ("Eroica"), during the years leading up to 1804 with Napoleon as the intended dedicatee. Through one of those fortuitous coincidences of fate, the news that Napoleon will crown himself Emperor arrives in Vienna as Beethoven prepares the title page of his symphony. In a fit of rage at this perceived betrayal of democracy, he tears the page in two, scratches out Napoleon's name, saying: "Then he too is nothing but an ordinary mortal! Now he also will tread all human rights underfoot, will gratify only his own ambition, will raise himself up above all others and become a tyrant!"[2]

The fifty-seven-year period that spanned Beethoven's lifetime (1770–1827) was one of unprecedented social and political turmoil. In no period of history – until the twentieth century – had so many events affected so many people in so many countries in so short a time. The eighteenth century in Europe is commonly called the Age of Enlightenment. A spirit of questioning, enquiry, and discovery animated all spheres of knowledge. New frontiers in the sciences were breached, and fundamental beliefs, such as the existence of God and the authority of church and state, were questioned. Major developments in the natural sciences, and to a lesser extent in biology and medicine, reflected this thinking. Regrettably, this enlightened attitude did not modify man's behaviour: this period saw wars, revolts, and humanitarian disasters as ugly as any in history.

The Enlightenment also spawned dramatic developments in art, literature, and especially in music. During the Enlightenment, generally regarded as ending with the onset of the French Revolution in 1789, J.S. Bach, Handel, Rameau, Haydn, and Mozart, among many others, composed their great music. The end of this innovative era coincided with the beginning of Beethoven's compositional career, but his formative years were spent at the height of the Enlightenment, and he was much influenced by both the music and the philosophy of the period.

A brief account of the momentous political events that took place in Western Europe during Beethoven's lifetime will provide a contextual background to his life and music. Knowledge of this background is helpful to understanding Beethoven's creativity because he had an active interest in these events and in the social and philosophical undercurrents that had led up to them, and they had a profound impact on his music and his compositional career. The state of knowledge in health and medicine during that epoch illuminates the attitude of Beethoven's physicians towards his health problems and illustrates the treatments to which he likely was subjected.

THE POLITICAL SCENE

The German-speaking areas of central Europe during the eighteenth century were divided into about three hundred semi-autonomous principalities, the majority ruled by an autocratic and hereditary prince, king, or archbishop. The principalities were loosely linked into an organization called the Holy Roman Empire, which had been established by Charlemagne in C.E. 800 with the Emperor in Vienna as its titular head. Intense rivalry between the two most powerful principalities, Austria and Prussia, continued well into the mid-nineteenth century, ending in a war won by Prussia.

One of the intriguing issues in eighteenth-century music history concerns the factors that favoured the development of Vienna as the musical capital of Europe, despite the fact that it was a much smaller centre than London, Paris, or Naples. Vienna's musical reign began with the accession of Ferdinand II to the throne in 1619.[3] As Emperor, Ferdinand encouraged links between the court and musicians from Italy and other countries, hence it became receptive to musical ideas. Through the seventeenth and eighteenth centuries both the court and generations of aristocratic families such as the Esterhazys and the Lichnowskys poured money into music, and a middle-class musical audience who were prepared to pay to listen to good music also emerged.[4] The process was assisted by a long and strong tradition of folk and gypsy music in the regions of Europe ruled by the Empire. Leading musicians, including Haydn and Mozart, made Vienna their home, giving it a musical lustre, and the city became a magnet for ambitious young musicians such as Beethoven.

One of the principalities ruled by archbishops was the territory of Cologne, which included Bonn, the birthplace of Beethoven. Religiously governed states such as Cologne were known chiefly for their powerful sponsorship of the arts, particularly music. Funding for choirs and orchestras, artists and architects, created a flowering of music, painting, and architecture in their realms such as few societies had seen. Many eighteenth-century composers, including Bach, Haydn, and Mozart, held appointments to royal or princely courts as organists, instrumentalists, or *Kapellmeisters* – the term used to describe the musical director or conductor of a court orchestra. These highly sought-after positions provided the holders with financial security, in return for which they composed, performed, entertained, and even taught music to their royal employers. This patronage system is the likely reason why musicians and composers in Germanic countries sprouted like lilies in springtime during the seventeenth and eighteenth centuries. However, it also made composers dependent on and beholden to their regal employers. Beethoven rebelled against this system and refused many offers to become a *Kapellmeister*. His decision led to financial insecurity but it also gave him sought-after freedom and acted, as he himself admitted, as a spur to compose. It can be said with some truth that Beethoven was the world's first free-enterprise composer.

In the late eighteenth century Bonn, a city of around 10,000 people, was the capital of the electorate of Cologne and hence the seat of the Archbishop of Cologne. This fact, together with its location on the banks of the Rhine, gave the city a key economic edge over its neighbours.[5] While there was much poverty, as in all European cities at that time, there also was a prosperous middle class involved in commerce and manufacturing. Most of the economic activity in the city centred on the archbishop's palace; the town was kept neat and clean and was ruled by an ecclesiastical court under the direction of the archbishop. Although the archbishop's rule was authoritarian, the men of the church of that period were devoted to music and the theatre, and lavished largesse on both artistic forms.[6] The ruler in 1770, the year of Beethoven's birth, was Maximilian Friedrich, whose government was, by contemporary standards, enlightened. He turned a large room of the palace into a concert hall where performances of concerts, opera, and theatre were provided by his own orchestra, choir, and actors. The artistic, theatrical, and musical atmosphere in Bonn was high quality, powerful, and pervasive.[7] Friedrich's successor to the throne, Maximilian Franz, provided a pivotal impetus to Beethoven's career (see chapter 2).

German thinkers and writers such as Immanuel Kant (1724–1804), Johann Wolfgang von Goethe (1749–1832), and Johann Schiller (1759–1805) developed strong followings. Beethoven had a high regard for each

of these writers. He adhered to Kant's philosophy of toleration and reconciliation as exemplified in his influential work *Kritik der reinen Vernunft*
(Critique of Pure Reason, 1781).[8] A copy of this work was on the shelf in
Beethoven's study and was auctioned after his death. Kant considered
that our knowledge must be based on logical concepts and experience,
that human experience was a synthesis of sense perception and understanding, and that both in turn, were regulated by the faculty of reason.[9]
Beethoven's affinity with Kant lay in his response, through his art, to the
same underlying experiential issues.[10] Kant's skeptical approach meant
that he was attacked by both those who believed in religion and those who
were against it, and his works were banned by King Maximilian Franz of
Prussia.

Goethe was the forerunner of the Romantic movement that swept
Europe during the nineteenth century, and had become famous for his
poetry and plays, the best known of which is *Faust*, a play in rhyme that
describes how Faust sells his soul to the devil in exchange for youth and
sensuality and pays the price for his bargain. Goethe also developed the
idea of the heroic genius, and through his writing provided an ultimate
esthetic meaning to the richness and variety of life.[11] A meeting between
Goethe and Beethoven in 1812 is discussed in chapter 2.

Schiller graduated in medicine but rapidly became disenchanted with
his practice as an army surgeon and devoted the rest of his life to writing
poetry and plays that had a strong revolutionary motif. Schiller sought an
objective definition of art that would underscore its ethical character, and
he attempted to integrate Kant's theories into an elevated concept of art
work.[12] There was close kinship between Schiller's ideas and Beethoven's
music. Beethoven admired both Goethe's and Schiller's writings and set
their poetry to music. Schiller's poem "Ode to Joy," a paean to universal brotherhood, became part of the final movement of Beethoven's Symphony no. 9 in D minor, op. 125 ("Choral").

During the eighteenth century the Italian peninsula was split into three
geographical and political entities: the Papal States occupied the area
around Rome, the king of Naples ruled the south, and the north was part
of the Austrian empire. Despite this political division, Italy had a power-

ful influence on the arts, particularly in music. Opera dominated Italian music in the eighteenth century, and Italian opera dominated Europe.[13] Many Italians regarded German music as decadent because it was not composed for the human voice. In 1758, Jean-Jacques Rousseau, the French philosopher, took part in an extended debate on the relative merits of Italian and French opera, and came down firmly on the side of the Italian.[14]

In Italian cities, the opera house was the centre of musical life and for Italian composers the proper function and purpose of music was to intensify the meaning and expression that were embodied in words. Two forms of opera evolved: *opera buffa* and *opera seria* (respectively comic and serious opera). *Opera buffa* particularly lent itself to innovative musical techniques that spread to other musical genres. Many Italian performers and composers – including Antonio Vivaldi (1678–1741), Dominico Cimarosa (1749–1801), and Luigi Boccherini (1743–1805) – travelled and settled in other parts of Europe, disseminating their knowledge and their distinctive Italian artistic flavour throughout Europe. Beethoven had contact with Italian musicians who settled in or were passing through Vienna, including Antonio Salieri (1750–1825) and Gioachino Rossini (1792–1868). The Italian community in Vienna, moreover, was not confined to musicians: Giovanni Malfatti, one of the illustrious physicians who treated Beethoven, was from Tuscany in northern Italy. His relationship with Beethoven and his treatment of Beethoven's health problems are discussed in chapter 3.

Unlike Germany and Italy, by the eighteenth century both France and England had been nation-states for centuries and had been involved in longstanding political and military rivalry. When the Seven Years' War between England and France, with their respective allies, ended in 1763, much of Europe was devastated. Although England was the main victor of this war, this victory was short-lived. The American War of Independence, which began thirteen years later in 1776, when Beethoven was six years old, resulted in the defeat of England and the creation of a new nation in the Americas. It was here that the ideas of liberty and democracy expressed in the Enlightenment received their first concrete expression.

France, defeated in the Seven Years' War, had supported the Thirteen Colonies in their revolt against England, but French satisfaction in the colonists' victory was also brief. Economic, social, and political tensions in French society had been building up for decades, and the very success of the Colonies' revolt helped to unleash forces that led to the French Revolution in 1789. No country was left untouched by the political shocks that followed.

The Enlightenment in Great Britain was led by scientists such as Joseph Priestley (1733–1804), Henry Cavendish (1731–1810), and William Herschel (1738–1822); by thinkers and writers such as David Hume (1711–1776), Adam Smith (1723–1790), and Samuel Johnson (1709–1784); and by artists such as Joshua Reynolds (1723–1792) and Thomas Gainsborough (1727–1788). Hume and Smith were to have a powerful effect on the development of Western society during the nineteenth and twentieth centuries: Hume because of his liberal political philosophy, and Smith because of his sponsorship of a laissez-faire economic doctrine. In *The Wealth of Nations*, published in 1776, by symbolic coincidence the year of the Declaration of American Independence, Smith championed free trade and saw enlightened self interest as being socially and economically beneficial.[15]

The French Revolution – the epochal event of this period – had a powerful impact on Beethoven's developing political attitudes because he was at an impressionable age, just eighteen, when the Revolution began. Three thinkers played a prominent part in setting the tone for the revolt: Jean-Jacques Rousseau (1712–1778), Voltaire (1694–1778), and Denis Diderot (1713–1784), and they, together with other French writers, as well as David Hume, who spent three years in Paris during the 1760s, came to be called "Les Philosophes."[16]

Rousseau was the most radical of Les Philosophes, and the only true republican; in his persuasive writings he proclaimed the need for individual freedoms within a republican system of government. His best-known work, *Du contrat social* – with its famous opening phrase "L'homme est né libre, et partout il est dans les fers" (Man is born free, but is everywhere enchained) – was published in 1762, and Rousseau's name and ideas were eulogized by the Revolutionaries in 1789. Rousseau was also an accomplished musician. He wrote a successful opera, *Le devin du village* (1752), published a *Dictionaire du musique* (1768), and wrote many of the music entries in *l'Encyclopédie*.[17] He helped make Paris a leading centre of music in the eighteenth century, especially in the field of publishing.[18]

Voltaire and *les Encyclopédistes*, led by Denis Diderot, echoed Rousseau's message in different ways. Voltaire (born François Marie Arouet) had a tempestuous youth during which he was twice arrested and confined in the Bastille for his antiroyalist views; he was also banished to England for two years. However, his subsequent fame rested on his plays and poetry, his knowledge of – and his friendship with – aristocrats and royalty, and on his affluence. Voltaire attacked the shams and hypocrisies of state and church; *Candide*, his literary masterpiece, is a satire on the convictions of political and religious faith. Probably because of his own unjust incarceration, he was also a champion of those who had been unjustly persecuted.[19] Diderot also spent a brief time in jail for his antigovernment views. On his release he began work on his monumental collaborative *Encyclopédie*, described as "the most famous of all experiments in the popularization of knowledge."[20] The final volume was published in 1765, although supplements appeared subsequently. *L'Encyclopédie* received a wide circulation and had a powerful impact on society and on politics of the day. Diderot also played a key role in the development of the novel as a form of artistic expression, as is exemplified in *Le neveu de Rameau*, a novel based on the eighteenth-century French composer Jean-Phillipe Rameau.[21]

Even Louis XV of France suspected that major changes in society were imminent, and is reputed to have said "Après moi, le déluge," before his death from smallpox in 1774. Weak leadership from his successor Louis XVI, losses at war, economic recession, and a recall of the States-General in 1789 ignited the revolutionary fuse.[22] The situation in France during the following ten years fluctuated between the expansive idealism expressed in the *Declaration of the Rights of Man* in 1789 at the one extreme and the Reign of Terror (1793–95) at the other, when tens of thousands of French men and women, including Louis XVI and Marie Antoinette, were executed on the guillotine. There followed a war between France and the rest of Europe, and the situation stabilized only in 1799. Despite horrific excesses, there were major positive results: the Revolution promulgated the rights of the individual against the state, it placed the final nail in the coffin of feudalism, and it marked the beginning of the end of an autocratic and hereditary system of governance that had existed in Europe for more than 1,200 years. Together with the political and constitutional developments that were taking place in Britain and the United States, the French Revolution helped to lay foundations for the democratic systems of government that developed during the nineteenth and twentieth centuries.

As noted above, Beethoven was one of many in Europe who initially greeted both the Revolution and Napoleon with enthusiasm. Napoleon was seen as one who had risen from the masses, bringing leadership and stability, and seemingly accomplishing the republican ideals of the Revolution. However, he squandered this support by introducing an imperial system of government and the trappings of a police state that resembled the autocratic kingdoms that he had replaced. By crowning himself emperor, Napoleon disowned republicanism, a political orientation that, at the time, was dear to Beethoven. History has borne out his angry rejection of Napoleon's assumption of dictatorial powers.

When the French army occupied Vienna during 1798–99, Beethoven met General Bernadotte, the French ambassador in Vienna. The general had a high regard for Beethoven and suggested that Beethoven compose a work in Napoleon's honour. Beethoven's Symphony no. 3 in E flat major, op. 55 ("Eroica"), was the result. It was Beethoven's original intention to dedicate the symphony to Napoleon: in a letter of 26 August 1804 addressed to his publishers Breitkopf and Hartel Beethoven stated, "The title of the symphony is really Bonaparte."[23] He changed his mind when he heard of Napoleon's intention to crown himself Emperor and instead dedicated the symphony to Prince Lobkovitz, one of his sponsors and admirers; Beethoven did, however, allow the published work to include the words "Per festeggiare il sovvenire d'un grand Uomo" (To honour the memory of a great man) on the title page. Despite the change in dedication, the *Eroica* was inspired by Napoleon and remains an "incomparable witness" to his early promise.[24] Although the audience at the premiere in 1805 was shocked by the length and dissonances of the work, the musical public rapidly grasped its greatness, and this symphony has been a favourite concert hall piece ever since.

Beethoven was involved in the musical side of the Congress of Vienna (1814–15) that decided the fate of Europe after the defeat of Napoleon. A concert held in his honour in November 1814 was attended by many of the heads of state attending the Congress, and Beethoven composed music especially for the occasion.[25] However, an eye-witness account notes that although some experts idolized him, "a far greater number" were unable to appreciate his music.[26] In his later years, Beethoven became progressively more anglophile. He saw the British constitution and society as more tolerant than others in Europe, and his music received early and strong recognition in England. But although he received many invitations to visit the country, he never made the journey.

The Congress of Vienna ended a turbulent period in European history that had lasted a generation. Under the baleful and reactionary influence of the Austrian foreign minister Count Metternich, the Congress restored the Bourbon monarchy in France in the person of Louis XVIII (a nephew of Louis XVI) and restored or entrenched similar autocratic regimes throughout Europe.[27] The freedom that had burst forth during the Revolution had been too brief – and too bloody – to encourage further experimentation down that avenue. It would take the industrial and educational revolutions of the nineteenth and twentieth centuries to overturn the older social and economic structures and values before democratic values took firm root.

SOCIAL ISSUES

Rigid social stratification was accepted as the norm in European societies during the eighteenth and early nineteenth centuries. The king, prince, bishop, or his advisors, made all political decisions. While there was a slowly expanding and increasingly prosperous middle class, the vast majority of the population was poor and underprivileged. There was no effective way for dissent to be expressed. Those who protested too loudly risked imprisonment, banishment, or both – as with Voltaire and Rousseau in France – or their writings were banned – as with Kant in Germany. This repression only increased the resentment of those excluded from decision making, so that when war, deprivation, and social unrest were added to the mix in the late eighteenth century, Europe was ripe for revolution.

The economies of late eighteenth-century European states were still heavily agrarian. Eighty percent or more of the population lived in the countryside as serfs, peasants, or landowners; the proportion varied from a low of around fifty percent in Holland to a high of ninety-five percent in Russia.[28] The time and energies of peasants were devoted to food production, primarily for themselves but also for those who lived in towns and cities, with many city dwellers moving to the countryside at harvest time. At the close of the eighteenth century the largest cities in Europe were London (pop. 860,000) and Paris (pop. 650,000), with Madrid and Naples close behind. Vienna had a population of about 200,000. Movement from the countryside to the city remained slow but steady throughout the eighteenth century and became a flood only in the nineteenth century with the Industrial Revolution. The transition of Beethoven's family from Belgian countryside through Bonn and then to Vienna over three generations reflects this trend. Since economies followed the laissez-faire doctrine, there were extremes of affluence and poverty, with few safety nets for the poor other than (usually religious) charities.[29]

The Wars of Religion that dominated the sixteenth and seventeenth centuries were over, but organized religion, representing both Catholicism and the Protestant faiths, remained influential throughout Europe during the eighteenth century, despite the assaults by Enlightenment philosophies, although these philosophies did improve the spirit of tolerance between Catholic and Protestant. The French Revolution also accomplished the final political emancipation of Jews in France (full civil rights were extended to them in 1791) and in Europe during the Napoleonic era.[30] Still, many social and economic barriers remained.

Beethoven died just prior to the start of the railway age. Travel during his lifetime moved at the speed and comfort of the horse, a style that had not changed much in two thousand years. The stagecoaches, drawn by four to six horses, that were the main form of transport between cities were slow, uncomfortable, and crowded. Accidents were frequent and there was no compensation insurance.[31] Beethoven made two trips between Bonn and Vienna via Munich, a distance of about 1,050 kilometres. He made his first journey, in 1787, by coach and the travel time was two weeks. For the second trip he took the post-chaise, a smaller and lighter vehicle than a coach that was the fastest means of public transport at the time; the trip took eight days. Each journey involved nightly stopovers at inns and guesthouses along the way. After settling in Vienna in 1792, Beethoven is known to have taken only one further extended journey: a concert tour in 1796 that took him to Prague, Leipzig, Dresden, and Berlin. He was a reluctant traveler but was also reluctant to say so explicitly. He received a number of attractive offers to visit England and would express great interest at first, but in the end would excuse himself, usually for reasons of health.

MEDICINE AND HEALTH

Medicine and health care during the late eighteenth century were slowly climbing out of the straitjacket imposed by the teachings of Galen (a second-century physician whose medical writings were regarded with almost religious reverence) that had inhibited progress for centuries. Life expectancy was still low (about thirty for both men and women), and infant and child mortality high; a newborn baby had a less than fifty percent probability of surviving to adulthood. Childhood diseases such as diphtheria, whooping cough, and measles took a heavy toll. Anatomy was by far the most advanced of the medical disciplines. Knowledge about physiology, pathology, and clinical medicine was not only limited but also distorted because it was based on false premises and lack of basic information. In Beethoven's day the causes of most diseases were unknown; although the microscope was in use, with the primitive staining techniques of the day, this new technology was of little value for histopathology or for tracing the connection between bacteria and disease. Physicians' limited clinical skills were based largely on the medical history and observation (inspection) of the patient. Other than feeling the pulse, physicians did not lay hands on their patients. The stethoscope, invented by René Laënnec (1781–1826) in 1816, caused a sea change in medical knowledge and clinical interpretation of bodily functions.

Although William Harvey's *De motu cordis*, an epic study of the heart and circulation of the blood had been published in 1628, more than 170 years previously, the capillary connection between the arterial and venous halves of circulation was based only on logic and speculation. The existence and function of the lymphatic system was beginning to be unraveled.[32] Although the stomach was known to produce acid, the process of digestion was thought to be analogous to putrefaction because the existence of intestinal enzymes was unknown. Body warmth was thought to be caused by friction resulting from limb and body movements, and the metabolic functions of organs such as the liver and the spleen were unknown, as was the function of the circulatory system in transmitting nutrients and hormones. However, a monograph on pathology published in 1793 noted an association between "common tubercles" of the liver and "those accustomed to drink spirituous liquors," male sex, and old age.[33] The liver in such persons was small and firm, and had a yellow "scirrhus" appearance, and there was "yellow water" in the abdominal cavity.

It was widely believed that bowel problems were the basis of all pathology and that diseases were transmitted from poisons and toxins originating in the blood. Although this approach had its origins in the seventeenth century, it owed much to the forceful writings of François Broussais (1772–1838), a Paris physician who recommended copious bloodletting for a wide variety of diseases.[34] Logical treatment consisted in removing the toxins through the use of emetics, purgatives, diaphoretics (drugs that stimulate sweating), and bloodletting. Treatment had to produce a visible release of "toxic" body fluids in order to be effective. The rationale for bloodletting was that the disease was caused by the accumulation of unnamed poisons in the blood that would be removed along with the blood; the greater the volume, the more toxin removed. Physicians were sometimes competitive as to who could remove the most blood without causing the demise of the patient.

Bloodletting as a treatment for disease had been practiced at least since Roman times, but it reached its zenith in the early nineteenth century. Bleeding was induced by venesection, by "cupping," or by the use of leeches. Then, as often now, England lagged behind advances on the continent. An article by an English physician published in 1819 stated that "General bloodletting has often failed in general diseases from the timid manner in which it was employed; and there is great reason to believe that local bloodletting, in local diseases, has not been carried out to an extent sufficient to ensure success, in numerous instances. Our continental brethren employ this kind of evacuation much more successfully than we do; therefore we shall be wise in taking a lesson and a hint from our rivals."[35] The author recommended twelve leeches to the jaw for toothache, thirty to the knee for gout, and thirty to the chest for pleurisy. In the same issue, the *Medico-Chirurgical Journal* editorialized, "It is a humiliating experience to perceive that some medical practitioners in the nineteenth century, of reputed talent and experience, are denouncing topical bleeding as useless and unnecessary. If the understanding of such practitioners be not under the absolute dominion of prejudice and erroneous reasoning, to the total preclusion of conviction, an instructive lesson would be afforded by a dispassionate reference to Johnson's *Influence of Tropical Climes*, or *The Atmosphere of the British Isles*. Either of these valuable productions would clearly exhibit the fallacy of their doctrines, and would set their judgments right, on a highly important topic of practice." Around this time leeches became scarce in England and had to be imported. The resulting drastic increase in price meant that the poor were unable to benefit from their use.

There were occasional voices of sanity in this cacophony of bleeding. Phillippe Pinel (1745–1826) adopted a skeptical attitude to bleeding therapy in his widely used textbook of medicine, which went through six editions between 1798 and 1816.[36] Across the Atlantic, Samuel Thomson (1769–1843), a peripatetic medical herbalist in the United States, describe a meeting in 1813 with Dr Barton, an eminent physician in Philadelphia: "I stated to him my opinion of the absurdity of bleeding to cure diseases, and pointed out its inconsistency, as the same method was made use of to cure a sick man as to kill a well beast … Their mode of treating yellow fever, I found to my astonishment, was to bleed twice a day for ten days. This absurd practice being followed by the ignorant classes of the faculty merely because it has been recommended by a great man has destroyed more lives than has ever been killed by powder or ball."[37] Thomson got into legal problems because of his unorthodox views, and was even imprisoned briefly for allegedly causing the death of a patient.

For unknown reasons, Beethoven never mentions bleeding therapy in his letters, but in a letter to Beethoven, written in 1807, Dr Johann Schmidt, his physician at the time, states: "From leeches we can expect no further relief."[38] In this letter, Dr Schmidt mentions Beethoven's headache, implying that leeches were used to relieve that symptom, but it is also conceivable that the leeches were used to treat his deafness, as bleeding was an accepted therapy for deafness at that time. As late as 1840, more than thirteen years after Beethoven's death, bleeding was recommended for deafness in a respected Scottish textbook.[39]

It is likely that the practice of homeopathy – the use of very small quantities of herbs and medication that became widespread in Germany under the influence of Samuel Hahnemann (1755–1810) – was provoked in part by an awareness of the failures of "heroic" treatment such as purgation and bloodletting, but it was the introduction of "numerical medicine" by Pierre Charles Alexandre Louis (1787–1872) that sounded the death knell of bleeding as a standard form of treatment for many diseases.[40] Unfortunately this development occurred a decade after Beethoven's death.

Another form of treatment that became fashionable in the early nineteenth century was "galvanism," or electrical stimulation. Luigi Galvani (1737–1798) had carried out experiments in electrophysiology and had discovered that the electrical stimulation of a nerve in a dissected frog caused muscle contraction. In 1802 it was found that the heart of a dead frog retained electrical excitability for fifteen hours, whereas that of a decapitated human being lasted for only four and a half hours. Devices (batteries, although not called such at the time) were developed for producing electric currents and were subsequently used for the purpose of treating a wide variety of diseases, including deafness, blindness, paralysis, pain, and insanity, and many cures were claimed. In the treatment of deafness, one electrode was placed on the ear and the other attached to a specially designed headdress. Beethoven received galvanic treatment for his deafness but with little success (see chapter 3). By 1818 Pinel was expressing skepticism as to the efficacy of galvanic treatment in medical disorders.[41]

Other standbys of medical treatment in the early nineteenth century were cold water effusions, bathing, topical blistering, and drugs, the study of which were then known as *materia medica*. A textbook on *Materia Medica* published in 1825 classified drugs into eight categories: emetics, cathartics, enemata, diaphoretics, diuretics, antilithics, enemogogues, and expectorants.[42] With the exception of antilithics, each of these categories stimulated a body secretion or excretion thought to be required for effective therapy. Opium and alcohol were widely used to relieve pain, particularly for surgical procedures. Bleeding was also used as an anesthetic, the surgery being performed once loss of consciousness had resulted from the blood loss. Chemical agents such as antimony and mercury were also used. Antimony was used as an emetic. Mercury was presented in powders, ointments, pills, and lotions, and was the treatment of choice for syphilis; in the form of mercury chloride ("Calomel") it was effective as a laxative. Its side effects on skin, teeth, and other organs were also well known.

"Animal magnetism" – what we now know as hypnosis – had a vogue before and during Beethoven's lifetime. This treatment was developed by Anton Mesmer (1734–1815), a Viennese physician who moved to Paris, where he created a sensation by curing diseases at séances. When he refused to reveal his secret, he was denounced by a special commission of the Paris Academy of Medicine. It is not known whether Beethoven underwent hypnosis for any of his medical problems, but with his assertive and skeptical personality, he would not likely have been a good hypnotic subject.

Treatment of the insane in pre-revolutionary Europe was primitive in the extreme and depended largely on restraint, punishment, and incarceration. One of the many landmark events of the French Revolution occurred in 1793, when Philippe Pinel, a leading Paris physician and a revolutionary, released the restraints of inmates confined at the Bicêtre Hospital.

This event dramatized the treatment of the mentally ill and inaugurated a more humane approach, which was powered by William Tuke (1732–1822) in England and by Johann Langermann (1768–1832) and Johann Christian Reil (1759–1813) in Germany. The onset of the Romantic movement in the early nineteenth century encouraged this development, and "treatment" gradually came to replace "punishment" in the management of insanity.[43] This change was given special impetus in England because of the periodic attacks of insanity experienced by George III (1738–1820), whose illness is now known to have been caused by porphyria, a genetically transmitted condition that can affect the brain. Small private homes or "pensions" were available for the residential treatment of those who could afford it, but more humane treatment of insanity in public facilities did not come until deep into the nineteenth century. Beethoven was fortunate that his psychiatric problems, although severe at times, did not require residential treatment.

The three major medical advances of the eighteenth century were the use of cowpox inoculations to provide immunity against smallpox, the use of "foxglove" (digitalis) to treat certain forms of "dropsy," and the use of citrus fruit to prevent scurvy. Smallpox had been the cause of death of up to twenty percent of the population. Inoculation (as distinct from vaccination), practiced since the early eighteenth century, consisted of applying a small quantity of the contents of the pustule from the skin of a person with smallpox to the scarified area of the skin of a healthy individual. The objective was to induce a milder form of smallpox, but in many cases the inoculated person became seriously ill. Edward Jenner (1749–1823), an English physician practicing in the countryside, learned that milkmaids who developed "cowpox" from an udder infection of the cows that they milked appeared resistant to smallpox. Jenner pondered this for some years before carrying out an experiment in which he gave cowpox to a young boy (a procedure that likely would have difficulty gaining the approval of present-day ethics review committees), and six weeks later applied pus from a smallpox victim. The child did not develop the disease. Jenner wrote up his results in a monograph,[44] and despite some initial resistance, inoculation rapidly became widespread in England and France; its use took longer to develop in Germany because of sustained opposition by a number of key individuals, including Immanuel Kant. The debate in Germany took the form of extensive philosophical and ethical discussions for and against inoculation and the decision, in the end, was largely left to individual enlightened physicians.[45] Beethoven's face was covered with pock marks and it is thought by some that he had smallpox as a child, but this is not known for certain; his condition may have been the result of severe acne.

In 1785 William Withering, a physician to the General Hospital in Birmingham, England, published a landmark study[46] on the medical use of foxglove in which he describes how his opinion was "awakened" by the success of an old woman in Shropshire who frequently cured "dropsy" when physicians' treatments had failed. Withering describes the use of foxglove (digitalis) in a series of 163 patients. At the time, dropsy was thought to be a unitary disease, but we now know that severe peripheral and abdominal edema (the condition that was then called dropsy) can be caused by several underlying disease processes, including primary cardiac, hepatic, and renal conditions. Digitalis is effective largely in the cardiac type, but not in other forms of the condition. It is interesting to note that even in Withering's case histories, foxglove was effective only in cardiac forms of the condition, although Withering himself did not recognize this distinction. Beethoven died of "dropsy," and it is very likely, although we do not know for certain, that he was given digitalis during his terminal illness. Because his disease was caused by a hepatic, rather than a cardiac, condition, the digitalis would not have been effective.

Scurvy was the curse of seamen during the sixteenth, seventeenth, and eighteenth centuries, and many thousands died painful deaths during long ocean voyages because of the lack of fresh fruit and vegetables in their diet. In 1753 James Lind (1716–1794), a Scottish physician with the Royal Navy, published his findings recommending lemon juice for the prevention and treatment of scurvy.[47] Unfortunately, many more sailors had to die before the Navy, forty-two years later, finally ordered lemons aboard all ships setting out on long voyages. While venereal disease was common, syphilis and gonorrhea were not recognized as separate diseases until the 1830s. Mercury preparations, the treatment of choice for these conditions, had limited efficacy and serious toxic effects. The use of mercury in the treat-

ment of syphilis was known as the scourge of Venus and Mercury, implying that the treatment was as harmful as the disease.[48] The controversy
about Beethoven's possible infection with syphilis is discussed in chapter
4. Tuberculosis was also common, particularly in crowded, unhygienic
areas of cities, and it took the lives of many, including Beethoven's mother,
his brother Carl, and possibly his infant sister, who died a few months
after his mother's death. Nothing was known about the cause or treatment
of tuberculosis in Beethoven's time.

The early nineteenth century saw the beginning of the application of
the scientific method to medical research. In 1800–01 François-Xavier
Bichat attempted to correlate clinical symptomatology with pathological
(autopsy) findings.[49] Some years later, Laënnec (1781–1826) introduced
the stethoscope,[50] and William Beaumont (1785–1853), a surgeon in the
American army, published a monograph on gastric physiology.[51]

The "hygiene" movement and "Brunonianism" had developed in the
medical community during the late eighteenth century, and both incorporated a theoretical structure for viewing health and disease and a practical
format for disease prevention and treatment. These movements existed
in England and France but were particularly powerful in Germany. The
hygiene movement was led by Pierre-Jean-Georges Cabanis (1757–1808)
in France[52] and by Christoph Wilhelm Hufeland (1762–1836) in Germany.[53] This movement emphasized the role of the environment in health
and illness and the importance of working with nature in the treatment of
disease. It was based on the Hippocratic tradition and dignified the role
of the physician in society. It also emphasized the importance of fresh air,
diet, exercise, and moderation in all things as an aid to health, as well as
"taking the waters" at health spas as treatment for many diseases.

Health spas had been used in medicine since antiquity but reached their
zenith in the eighteenth and early nineteenth centuries.[54] The eighteenth
century saw a rapid development in chemistry and chemical analysis, and
there was much debate about the chemical composition of water for drinking and bathing, its effect on health, and its uses in treatment of disease.[55]
Knowledge of the chemical constituents of water gave physicians confidence that their recommendations were based on scientific principles.
Water therapy was recommended for different diseases, including fevers,

burns, rheumatism, gout, and insanity, and involved a wide variety of procedures, including bathing or immersion in hot or cold water for short or
prolonged periods, showering, or jets of water on the affected body part.
Water therapy began to lose its appeal in the late nineteenth century with
major advances in scientific medicine, and by the mid-twentieth century
had been largely dropped from the treatment arsenal. Beethoven, following his doctor's orders, spent most summers of his adult life taking "cures"
at health spas around Vienna. He went to Baden most frequently, probably because it was only twenty-five kilometres from Vienna, but he also
spent time at Heilegenstadt, Teplitz, and Karlsbad. The waters at Baden
contained high levels of calcium, sulphates, and hydrogen sulphide and
were particularly recommended for rheumatological disorders.[56] Judging
from the comments made in his letters, Beethoven seems to have believed
strongly in the efficacy of water treatment.

The hygiene movement also encouraged exercise and fresh air, particularly walking in the country, as salubrious to health. A publication
in 1815 contains long chapters on these and related topics, such as diet,
nutrition, beverages (alcoholic and non-alcoholic), sleep, work, climate,
and "les passions," which include love and sexuality.[57] Although some of
these claims are exaggerated, the theme was moderation in all things, and
few statements are inconsistent with modern thinking on these topics.[58]

"Brunonianism" was less valid and enduring. The movement is named
for John Brown (1735–1788), a Scottish physician who described his ideas
in *Elementa Medicinae,* a book first published in Latin in 1780.[59] These
ideas were strongly taken up by Johann Erhard (1766–1827) and others in
Germany after 1795. Brunonianism attempted to bridge the gap between
theory and practice by presenting a unified system of medical practice.
It relied heavily on philosophical theory and attempted to integrate its
approach with the philosophy of Immanuel Kant. Brunonianism presup-
posed that life existed only when external stimuli impinged on matter
that possessed "irritability," and health existed when there was a balance
between the two forces of stimuli and matter. Illness resulted if this balance was upset by over- or understimulation, "sthenia" being caused by
overstimulation, and "asthenia" by understimulation. Treatment consisted of restoring this balance by means of exercise, diet, and medica-

tion; opium and brandy were used for diseases diagnosed as asthenic. Although the supporters of Brunonianism emphasized that illness was not the result of pathology and dysfunction of a part of the body, the treatment appeared to make sense because it attacked the presumed "cause" of the illness. Brunonianism provoked intense conflict and controversy in Germany. It was practiced and propagated particularly by younger physicians who were attempting a revolution against the medical establishment and the faculties of medicine in a medical equivalent to the political upheavals that were taking place in society as a whole, and it also reflected a generational conflict, as it was taken up by young physicians, while older physicians based in academic medical centres defended traditional medicine. However, Brunonianism lacked a theoretical grounding and a satisfactory practical base, in particular because the patient lost his/her individuality and became a mere receptacle for external stimuli. This, in the end, became its undoing and Brunonianism began to peter out as a force in medicine after 1815.

With his many health problems, Beethoven inevitably became involved in these various currents and controversies. Johann Peter Frank (1745–1821), his physician from 1800–09, was a professor in the faculty of medicine in Vienna, a famous physician, and a leading opponent of Brunonianism. Frank wrote a standard work on hygiene and public health that became very influential, in which he describes how a government could act to improve the health of its subjects.[60] He and Beethoven's later physicians were instrumental in encouraging the composer's annual summer pilgrimages to the springs and spas around Vienna, and, judging from Beethoven's comments in his letters, these treatments were effective in improving his sense of well-being and also stimulating his creativity. In May 1825 Beethoven wrote a long letter to Anton Braunhofer, his physician at the time.[61] This letter is a fascinating example of written role play in which he describes his symptoms and pleads for changes in treatment, gently but firmly asking his doctor to recommend Brown's approach, which had previously been denied.

Esteemed Friend!
Doctor: How are you, my patient?

Patient: We are rather poorly – we still feel very weak and are belching and so forth. I am inclined to think that I now require a stronger medicine, but it must not be constipating – surely I might be allowed to take white wine diluted with water, for that poisonous beer is bound to make me feel sick – my catarrhal condition is showing the following symptoms, that is to say, I spit a good deal of blood, but probably only from my windpipe. But I have frequent nose bleedings, which I often had last winter as well. And there is no doubt that my stomach has become dreadfully weak, and so has, generally speaking, my whole constitution. Judging by what I know of my own constitution, my strength will hardly be restored unaided.

Doctor: I will help you. I will alternate Brown's method with that of Stohl.

Patient: I should like to be able to sit at my writing desk again and feel a little stronger. Do bear this in mind – Finis.

I will look you up as soon as I go into town. Just tell Karl at what time I can find you. But it would help me if you could inform Karl what other remedies I should use. The last medicine you prescribed I took only once and then lost it – With kindest regards and my gratitude, Your friend Beethoven

He also enclosed a brief canon addressed to the doctor, the text of which reads: "Close the door against Death, I plead, Doctor, notes will help in need." The "notes" are presumably the musical notes of the canon.[62] Although we do not have Dr Braunhofer's response, it seems unlikely that he was agreeable to changing his treatment approach to one toward which he had strong philosophical objections.

CULTURE AND POLITICS

Art and culture reflect the society in which they are created. The French Revolution and its aftermath had a profound effect on Beethoven and on his creativity, and the political turmoil also affected other artists of his generation. The character of Beethoven's music has its origins in the music of the French Revolution. According to Frida Knight, "Beethoven was part of history in the making ... one cannot understand him in humanitarian and social terms if one knows nothing of the impulses that went to make the

French Revolution."[63] Knight states that the historical events of the 1790s – revolution, class war, the war between France and the rest of Europe that culminated in Napoleon's rise to power and his victories against all odds – stimulated creativity in artists and composers in part because of the admiration and adulation, even if misplaced and temporary, that these events aroused. Despite his friendships with many aristocrats, and his initial claim of aristocratic descent (because of the "van" prefix in his surname), Beethoven regarded himself as a republican. He supported the revolutionary Declaration of the Rights of Man and had a lifelong admiration for the revolutionary ideals of liberty and brotherhood.[64] However, according to Anton Schindler (1795–1864), Beethoven's secretary in his final years, these republican sympathies moderated somewhat later in life when he became acquainted with the British constitution.[65] Schindler states that Beethoven's political views were based on the philosophies of Plato and Plutarch, that they were republican and democratic, and that Beethoven had admired Napoleon in the early years because he drew order out of chaos. Schindler also notes that Beethoven could be very indiscreet in expressing his political views. His basic political conception was the right of the individual to liberty and personal development.

Beethoven did not belong to any political organizations but he took a lively interest in current events. In his later years he was frequently and loudly critical of the autocratic Austrian regime of Metternich.[66] Metternich was chancellor of Austria for more than thirty years, beginning in 1815, and his regime had all the trappings of a police state, with paid informers, secret police, and imprisonment without trial,[67] but Beethoven was never hounded or pursued, likely in part because of his international fame but also because of his patent lack of political organizational skills.

Beethoven had designated Johann Rochlitz (1769–1842) – a friend and admirer, who was also one of the best known writers on musical topics in the early nineteenth century – to be his biographer but Rochlitz declined the honour, ostensibly because he was overworked.[68] Rochlitz described Beethoven's behaviour in a group at a tavern in 1822, talking loudly, monopolizing the conversation, and expressing strong political views that were full of admiration for England and extremely critical of France:

"[Beethoven] impressed me as being a man with a rich aggressive intellect, an unlimited, never resting imagination."[69] Friedrich Kanne, a leader at the time of student uprisings in Vienna in 1817–18, was a frequent visitor to Beethoven and "communicated his fiery indignation to the conversation books."[70] Knight gives fascinating examples of political discussions from Beethoven's Conversation Books: "His friends often took Beethoven out to eat, or to his favourite beerhouses; but the shadows of the ubiquitous secret police were apt to dampen conviviality. Beethoven himself did not care who heard his opinions, but his companions did not want to be arrested for subversion, so we find Oliva (a friend) shushing him up, and Karl (his nephew) writing 'Silentium! Die Stöcke haben Ohren!' (Silence! The walls have ears!)."[71] On another occasion in the tavern, a suspicious character was hovering nearby. To Beethoven's query as to who it was, Oliva replied "Police in disguise, prowling around ... he is dressed up as a military ... it is all part of the Inquisition." There is an incident and a gendarme removes one of the customers. "The one in blue asked his name," Oliva writes, "and then said he had orders to arrest him; so the other resisted him, and then the first man called the one in grey, a police sergeant, and he arrested him and took him away."

An interesting interchange from 1826 is recorded in the Conversation Books between Beethoven and Grillparzer, a well-known poet who nine months later was to write Beethoven's funeral oration. Grillparzer writes: "The Censor has assassinated me," and after Beethoven's (unrecorded) reply, adds, "One has to go to North America to give free expression to one's thoughts."[72]

In November 1820 Beethoven had a visit from Dr Miller, a philologist from the German town of Bremen, who commented on his outspoken interest in all that was happening. "His sense of cosmopolitan independence ... might have been the reason why, over and over again he continued a conversation begun earlier, and expressed opinions freely and candidly about everything, the government, the police, the manners of the aristocracy, in a critical and mocking manner."[73] Knight concludes that "the very fact that the battle was being waged, that people still had the courage, the heroism, the passion enabling them to fight for freedom, aroused Beethoven's own courage and passion; and this is one of the reasons why 1820 is one of the years in which he was able to write such great and human music as the last three piano sonatas and the Diabelli Variations through which the revolutionary wind breathes and blows, sometimes rising to gale force."

The music of the revolution, including "La Marseillaise," which became the French national anthem, had a powerful effect on the development of Beethoven's second period music,[74] but his most profound political statement is his Symphony no. 9, op. 125, written in the shadow of the Congress of Vienna that re-established autocratic and reactionary regimes throughout Europe. Among its themes, taken from Schiller's poem, "Ode to Joy," are brotherly love, hope, and individuality, all of which were antithetical to post-Napoleonic Europe. This message was not lost on the enthusiastic audiences who applauded its performances. The symphony provided people with an outlet for their political frustration. Lockwood has discussed the political implications of the ninth symphony in detail, and he sees this work, together with the *Missa solemnis*, as symbolizing respectively Beethoven's secular and religious philosophies.[75] Buch has described how, during the twentieth century, the Symphony no. 9 was appropriated by political organizations ranging from National Socialism to Communism, and he notes that the setting of Schiller's "Ode to Joy" in the fourth movement, which was used as the anthem of the racist regime of Rhodesia in the 1970s, is now the anthem of the European Union.[76]

While composing music that was striking in its originality and beauty, Beethoven was also, by his life experiences, a child of his times. He was able to bring the passion and intensity of the revolutionary changes taking place in society during his lifetime to his music. The continued popularity of his music shows that it can transcend the boundaries of time and of social and political ideologies. Through his natural talent and his "uninterrupted diligence," Beethoven was able, as Count Waldstein had foretold, to receive and extend Mozart's genius.

CHAPTER TWO

Beethoven's Life

"I shall seize Fate by the Throat; it shall certainly not crush and bend me completely."

Beethoven to Franz Wegeler, 1801[1]

Beethoven's life was filled with incident. He had a hard-driving, extroverted nature and made things happen. To use a modern term, he was a "mover and shaker." Even apart from his music, his life and character have fascinated biographers. In this chapter I will discuss his family background and the main events of his life, with an emphasis on his health and his relationships with family and friends, and in particular with women. Although not all of these relationships are connected with his health, they were often intense and stormy, and they provide us with an intriguing glimpse of his personality. His musical compositions will be mentioned only in these contexts.

Many musicologists have divided Beethoven's music into three distinctive periods or styles: the early (classical), the middle (heroic), and the late (mature).[2] There has been criticism of this categorization. Most significantly, it ignores the music that Beethoven composed in Bonn, before moving to Vienna. Kinderman acknowledges the historic relevance of the three "Vienna" styles, but further divides each one into two, or even three sub-categories, and identifies the final five "Galitzen" quartets as a category of their own.[3] A critique of this debate is outside the scope of this book. The following biographical sketch is structured around Beethoven's family background and four musical periods: one in Bonn and three in Vienna.

FAMILY BACKGROUND

Beethoven's grandfather (also called Ludwig) immigrated to Bonn in the 1730s from the area around Malines in the Flemish part of what is now Belgium.[4] Beethoven himself made few references to his Flemish origins, although he is thought to have visited the area with his mother around the age of eleven. Claims have been made that many of his traits, attitudes, and ideals, his independence and passionate love of liberty, and his treatment of the nobility as equals are more consistent with the Flemish than the Germanic character of the period.[5] His Flemish ancestry also explains the "van" (rather than the German "von") that prefixes the family name. In Flanders "van" did not have the connotation of aristocratic ancestry that it had in Germany. It has also been suggested that the name "Beethoven" is derived from the word "*beet*," the Flemish word for beetroot, indicating a family connection with beetroot farming. After an investigation into the origin of "van Beethoven" Thayer concluded that since the "*van*" is the Flemish word for "from," it is more probable that the name referred to Bethouvre, a small town in Belgium, indicating that the family was "from Bethouvre."[6]

Ludwig (senior) had had voice training and because of his musical talents was invited by the archbishop of Cologne to come to Bonn, initially as a musician and later as *Kapellmeister*. An older brother, Cornelius, was already living in Bonn and their father, Michael, who was attempting to flee from bankruptcy creditors, followed them.[7] Ludwig was an excellent musician, and he is also alleged to have been a composer, although none of his works have survived. Later in life he developed a business sideline trading in wine. His wife, Josepha, had an alcohol problem and because of this spent much of the latter part of her life in a cloister. The couple's only sur-

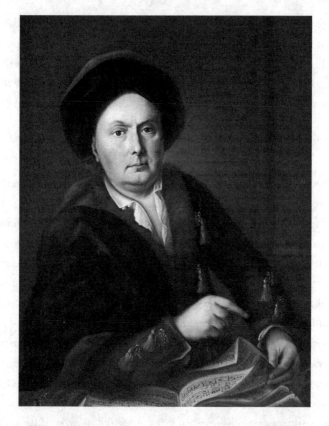

Ludwig van Beethoven (1712–1773), the composer's grandfather,
who died when Beethoven was three years old. Beethoven revered his grandfather
and kept this picture throughout his life. Beethoven-Haus, Bonn.

viving child, Johann, was to become Beethoven's father. Ludwig became
Beethoven's godfather, but he died in 1773 when Beethoven was three
years old. Although he had few memories of his grandfather, Beethoven
had a high regard for him, and during his childhood would encourage his
mother to tell him stories about the old man.[8] When Beethoven moved to
Vienna he took with him a portrait of his grandfather that remained in his
possession until he died.

Much of what we know about Beethoven's childhood and home comes from Gottfried Fischer (1780–1864), a friend and neighbour of the family who at age sixty wrote down his memories of their household.[9] Fischer described the home of the grandparents as "beautiful and well arranged." Beethoven's father, Johann, had a limited education and was described as "distinguished in neither intellect nor morals."[10] He was well trained as a musician, particularly as a vocalist, and was employed as such by the elector, the archbishop of Cologne. However, he had an unstable temperament, and in the mid-1770s developed an alcohol problem that caused further behavioural instability. Family conflicts, illnesses, and deaths forced Beethoven to mature at a young age. His reaction to an incident that occurred when he was eighteen reflects this early maturity. The police arrested Beethoven's father when intoxicated, and the young man was required to bail him out of prison; as a result, Johann lost his position in the choir and hence his income. Beethoven wrote to the elector asking that he be awarded the allowance that had previously gone to his father. Although Beethoven's letter of application is not available, the elector's positive response is extant.

Maria Magdalena, Beethoven's mother, came from a respectable family in the Moselle and Rhine regions of Germany, whose members included generations of councilors, clergy, and civil servants. In 1767, when she married Johann, she was already a widow who had lost an infant son in her first marriage. Fischer describes her as a "good domestic woman," but one who rarely laughed and was made gloomy by the vicissitudes of life.[11] According to other descriptions of her character she was "always serious" and rarely laughed; she was pious and gentle, but could be "vehement" in conflicts within the family. She was also described as a "quiet, suffering woman." Although Beethoven later in life spoke of her as an "excellent" mother, it appears likely that she provided him with little affection and protection, initially because of her melancholic disposition and later because of her poor health. Maria-Magdalena developed tuberculosis and died from this condition in 1787 when Beethoven was not yet seventeen. Johann died in 1792, likely from the complications of alcoholism, shortly after Beethoven left Bonn to settle in Vienna.

THE BONN PERIOD

Johann and Maria-Magdalena's first child, Ludwig Maria, born in 1769, lived only six days. The fact that this was the second infant she had lost may be one reason for her emotional detachment from her second child of this marriage, the young Beethoven, who was born in December 1770. There is uncertainty about his exact birthdate. An extant baptismal certificate for 17 December 1770 does not give a date of birth, but because of the high infant mortality rate at the time, it was the Catholic custom to baptize newborn infants within a day or two of birth; this was even more probable given that the family had already lost an infant son the previous year. It is likely, therefore, that Beethoven was born on 15 or 16 December 1770, with the latter date being the more likely. Another curiosity is that until his mid-forties Beethoven believed that he had been born in 1772. His father deliberately falsified his son's age in order to better promote him as a child prodigy: an extant advertisement of Beethoven's first public performance in 1778 gives Beethoven's age as six. Maria Magdalena gave birth to three more living children: Caspar Carl in 1774, Nikolaus Johann in 1776, and a daughter, Maria Margaretha Josepha, who was born in May 1786 but died in November 1787 at the age of eighteen months, likely from tuberculosis, shortly after her mother's death.

Beethoven attended the local primary school and completed basic courses in writing and arithmetic, but from an early age his father promoted his training in music, this also being consistent with his natural aptitudes. His music studies led to a neglect of his general education and, as a result, he never proceeded to the gymnasium (high school). For the rest of his life he remained relatively deficient in grammar and arithmetic. However, he did learn Latin and French, and his command of written French was good enough for him to write letters in French to correspondents in England, Scotland, Sweden, and Russia. During his teens he attended philosophy courses at the University of Bonn, and he kept works of Plutarch, Homer, and Kant in his personal library. He read widely in the arts, poetry, and philosophy and was self-educated in these areas. Fischer describes him as a "shy and taciturn" boy, but also as mischievous and not beyond playing practical jokes.[12] He appears to have been a "loner" as a child and to have had a vivid imagination, particularly when exposed to music and poetry.

Beethoven's musical education began at age four with his father, who used threats and punishments: examples given by Fischer when Ludwig was at the piano include, "What silly trash are you scratching together again now?" and "What are you splashing around for; go away or I'll box your ears." Despite this, young Ludwig progressed rapidly, and Johann finally came to praise his excellence and predict his success. Beethoven's first public performance was in 1778 when he was eight, but nothing is known of the reception. Beethoven reportedly told Carl Czerny, "I received harsh treatment and insufficient instruction from my father, but I had a talent for music."[13]

Christian Neefe, the cathedral organist, became Beethoven's teacher when the boy was nine, and by age eleven, he was able to replace Neefe as organist. The latter was not only a good teacher; Beethoven "never had a warmer, kinder and more valuable friend" than Neefe.[14] When Beethoven was thirteen Neefe wrote, "He would surely become another Mozart were he to continue as he had begun."[15]

Beethoven's lifelong relationship with the von Breuning family began in 1784 when his friend Franz Wegeler introduced him to this household.[16] The family consisted of the mother, Helene, and her four children: Eleonore (called "Lorchen"), thirteen at the time, Christoph, age eleven, Stephan, age nine, and Lorenz (called "Lenz"), age seven. Their father, Emanuel Joseph, had died in a fire in the archbishop's palace during the winter of 1776–77 while attempting to save important documents. Hélène, rather than wearing "widow's weeds,"[17] more than compensated for the traumatic loss of her husband, both as a model mother and by making her house the intellectual centre of the leading citizens of Bonn. She also became Beethoven's surrogate mother. During his teenage years Beethoven spent many days and even nights at the von Breuning home, and Hélène had a strong formative influence on his character and his education. According to Wegeler, "Friends of the house excelled in the sort of sociable entertainment that unites usefulness with pleasure."[18] Wegeler added that Beethoven felt free when he was with the von Breunings; he moved around the house with ease and this atmosphere made him cheerful and developed his mind. In 1825 Wegeler, who eventually married Eleonore von Breuning, wrote to Beethoven, "My mother-in-law's home was more your residence than your own."[19] Beethoven certainly needed this positive influence, given the increasingly distressing circumstances of his own family arising from his alcoholic father and tuberculotic mother. Hélène von Breuning had a generous and understanding way of dealing with Beethoven's sometimes difficult behaviour and would exonerate him by saying, "He is having a raptus again." She likely knew the origin of this term as the Latin word for "seizure," suggesting uncontrolled behaviour. Beethoven continued to use the expression in later life to describe, and perhaps justify, some of his periodic emotional or behavioural problems.[20] In later life Beethoven referred to the von Breuning family as his guardian angels and said that Frau von Breuning "knew how to keep insects away from the blossoms."[21] She filled the void in his heart left when his mother died in 1787, and then broadened his education by introducing him to the classics, poetry, and German literature.

The four von Breuning children all had successful careers. Beethoven became very fond of Eleonore, and she likely was his first love while he was a teenager visiting the household in Bonn. She was four months younger than he, and was one of the signatories of the Zehrgarten Stammbuch given to Beethoven in 1792 on his departure for Vienna. Her entry in the Stammbuch is a brief quotation from a poem by Johann Herder: "'Friendship with one who is good grows like the evening shadows until the sun of life sets.' [signed] Your true friend Eleonore Breuning."[22] Two letters that Beethoven wrote to her after moving to Vienna indicate that they likely had a deeper relationship. The first letter, written in November 1793,[23] is affectionate. Beethoven refers to a quarrel they had had, but does not provide details, and he adds: "I would give a great deal to be able to blot out my behaviour which did me so little honour and which was inconsistent with my usual character ... the sincerest repentance is only to be found when the criminal himself confesses his crime and this is what I have wanted to do." In this letter, he enclosed a dedication to Eleonore of a piece that he had composed. She in turn sent him a neck cloth as a gift. His reply, written in June 1794,[24] states: "Your generous behaviour made me feel ashamed ... your remembrance made me tearful and sorrowful ... this loss [of their friendship] cannot and will not be made good very quickly." Although we will never know the cause of the initial rupture in their relationship, there seem to be two possibilities: one is that he was aggressive and lost his temper or threatened her; the other is that he was sexually importunate and she rejected him. After his departure for Vienna she and Beethoven never saw each other again, although they exchanged further letters of friendship and affection at the end of Beethoven's life. Wegeler became a physician and then rector of the University of Bonn. Beethoven continued to correspond with him after moving to Vienna, and valued his medical opinion. When he first became aware of the serious and progressive nature of his deafness in 1801, Beethoven wrote two emotional and appealing letters to Wegeler, vividly describing the trauma he was experiencing.[25]

Eleonore's brother Christoph von Breuning became a lawyer, and eventually a privy councilor in Berlin. Stephan, his younger brother, also became a lawyer and moved to Vienna where he and Beethoven shared living quarters for a time, but their relationship ruptured after an argument in 1804.[26] Although they maintained some contact, it was not until a year or so before Beethoven's death that a stable reconciliation occurred. In his will Beethoven left Stephan many of his personal possessions and, most importantly, the custody of his nephew Karl. Unfortunately, Stephan died unexpectedly only two months after Beethoven's death. Stephan's son Gerhard, who was thirteen at the time of Beethoven's death, visited Beethoven almost daily during the composer's final illness, bringing a shaft of light and gaiety into Beethoven's sombre life. Gerhard subsequently became a physician, and wrote a fascinating account of his memories of Beethoven.[27] Lorenz, the youngest of the four von Breuning children, also studied medicine but died unexpectedly at age twenty-one, shortly after graduating. Beethoven had a close friendship with Lorenz,

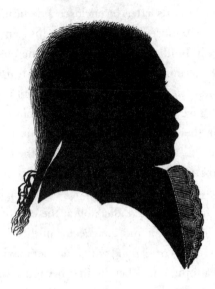

Silhouette of Beethoven, age sixteen, about a year before his first visit to Vienna, created by Joseph Neeson (1770–1829). Beethoven wears a wig and a lace-trimmed neckerchief, part of the mandatory costume in the court of the Archbishop elector of Bonn. Beethoven-Haus, Bonn.

and in a letter to Ferdinand Ries in 1804, wrote: "I have found only two friends in the world with whom, I may say, I have never had a misunderstanding. But what fine men! One is dead, the other is still alive."[28]

The von Breunings strongly promoted Beethoven's musical education. His earliest known compositions date from his teenage years, when he was still under the tutelage of Neefe: the Variations for Piano on a March by Dressler, WoO 63, a set of three piano sonatas (E flat major, F minor, and D major, WoO 47) – written in 1782 when Beethoven was twelve – and several short works written over the next three or four years. By age sixteen Beethoven realized that if he wished to develop his musical career, he needed to leave Bonn. With the probable financial assistance of Elector Maximillian Franz, Beethoven made the long trip by coach to Vienna, arriving in April 1787. During his two-week stay, he may have met both the Emperor Joseph and Wolfgang Amadeus Mozart.[29] Whether Beethoven had intended to remain in Vienna for a longer period is not known, but he likely returned early because of his mother's illness. He returned to Bonn by way of Munich and she died on 17 July 1787, shortly after his return. Beethoven's first extant letter, dated 15 September 1787 and addressed to an advocate, Dr Joseph von Schaden, whom Beethoven had met while passing through Augsberg on his return from Vienna, eloquently describes his mother's death, and the effect it had on his health.

I must confess that as soon as I left Augsberg my good spirits and my health too began to decline. For the nearer I came to my native town, the more frequently did I receive from my father letters urging me to travel more quickly than usual, because my mother was not in very good health. So I made as much haste as I could, the more so as I myself began to feel ill. My yearning to see my ailing mother once more swept all obstacles aside so far as I was concerned, and enabled me to overcome the greatest difficulties. I found my mother still alive, but in the most wretched condition. She was suffering from consumption and in the end she died about seven weeks ago after enduring great pain and agony. She was such a good, kind mother to me and indeed my best friend. Oh! Who was happier than I, when I could still utter the sweet name of mother it was heard and answered: and to whom can I say it now? To the dumb likenesses of her which my imagination fashions for me? Since my return to Bonn I have as yet enjoyed very few happy hours. For the whole time I have been plagued with asthma (*Engbrustigkeit*); and I am inclined to fear that this malady may even turn to consumption. Furthermore, I have been suffering from melancholia, which in my case is almost as great a torture as my illness.[30]

This letter, written less than two months after his mother's death, indicates that Beethoven was going through a profound bereavement reaction that not only affected his mood ("*melancholia*") but also gave him respiratory symptoms (*Engbrustigkeit* is translated as "asthma" by Anderson and as "tightness of the chest" by Marek)[31] that were likely similar to those experienced by his mother before her death. Since there is no further mention of lower respiratory tract problems in Beethoven's correspondence until

1816, it seems probable that he was experiencing hyperventilation symptoms that are easily mistaken for asthma; such symptoms may be provoked by anxiety and are common during bereavement.

Beethoven's words, "To whom can I say it [mother] now?" are curious, given her lack of availability to him through most of her lifetime, and suggest that he may have idealized her despite her apparent lack of affection. His continuing friendship with the von Breuning family indicates that Frau von Breuning likely helped him to work through his bereavement and filled a maternal role for him. To further compound his grief at this time, his infant sister died only two months later, possibly also from tuberculosis contracted from her mother. His father's continuing alcohol problems and the illnesses and deaths of his mother and sister left the family penniless. One of the people who provided help for the family at this stage was Ferdinand Ries's father.[32] Ries subsequently became one of Beethoven's best-known pupils, and Beethoven was eternally grateful to him for the assistance his father had rendered the Beethoven family when they were destitute.

Beethoven remained in Bonn for five and a half more disconsolate years. His father's descent into alcoholism accelerated (it was during this period that he was arrested and could no longer carry out his musical functions), and he died in 1792 shortly after Beethoven's departure for Vienna. In later life Beethoven spoke of his mother with affection but rarely mentioned his father.[33] His happiest times were spent with the von Breuning family, with his friends at a tavern known as the Zehrgarten, and wandering alone in the countryside around Bonn. There are no further direct references to health issues during the Bonn period, but in a long letter to Franz Wegeler written from Vienna in 1801, Beethoven indicates that he experienced other health problems while in Bonn.[34] He tells his friend (who by now was a physician) about the onset of his hearing loss, adding, "The trouble [deafness] is supposed to be caused by the condition of my abdomen which, as you know, was wretched even before I left Bonn, but has become much worse in Vienna, where I have been constantly afflicted with diarrhea and have been suffering in consequence an extraordinary debility." Although this is the first mention of gastrointestinal problems it is clear that it was already a chronic disorder that had started in his teens.

Beethoven's compositions dating from this five-year period in Bonn are mainly short pieces without opus numbers (WoO) that Thayer calls "trifles,"[35] but there are two more substantial works: the *Cantata on the Death of the Emperor Joseph II*, WoO 87 (1790) and the Octet, op. 103, scored for two oboes, two clarinets, two horns, and two bassoons, which was likely composed in 1792 although it was discovered only after his death. Beethoven established his reputation above all as a pianist, and his ability to improvise became legendary. Neefe stated in 1793 that he was "beyond controversy one of the foremost pianoforte players."[36]

By 1792, Beethoven and his friends in Bonn began to think that another visit to Vienna was required. The immediate rationale for the trip was to take lessons with Joseph Haydn, the leading composer of the day. Haydn had passed through Bonn early in the year on his return from London and had met and been impressed by Beethoven. The elector provided funding for the trip with the promise to send more money after Beethoven's arrival in Vienna. As noted above, his friends held a farewell party for the young composer at the Zehrgarten, and fourteen of them wrote farewell messages that provide a revealing insight into his relationships.[37] He likely took his leave with the intention of returning, and this was certainly his friends' expectation, but he never saw his native city again.

THE FIRST VIENNA (CLASSICAL) PERIOD

When Beethoven arrived in Vienna early in November 1792 the political situation was in a state of ferment, both in the countryside he travelled through and in Vienna. Reverberations of the French Revolution were felt throughout Europe, Franz II had just been crowned Holy Roman Emperor, and the country was preparing for an anticipated war with France. In Vienna, a capital city with a cosmopolitan population, the authorities kept close tabs on "foreigners" such as Beethoven.

After finding lodgings, his next two objectives were to buy a piano and set up visits and lessons with Joseph Haydn. Outwardly, the lessons were not as successful as had been anticipated. The complex and ambivalent relationship between Haydn and Beethoven has been a subject of major debate.[38] Both were strong-minded individuals, conscious of their capabilities as composers. Beethoven, a young, hardworking, creative, and ambitious musician, was relatively unknown at that time. Haydn, on the other hand, was at the zenith of his career and much in demand as a composer and teacher. He recognized Beethoven's exceptional talent and gave him encouragement. Beethoven was nonetheless critical of his teacher and questioned, among other things, Haydn's lack of attention to detail. It is clear from his music, however, that Beethoven owed a considerable debt to his erstwhile teacher. Beethoven also had lessons from Johann Albrechtberger (who was widely recognized as a teacher and a leading contrapuntalist), Antonio Salieri, and Johann Schenk, and developed a reputation as a difficult pupil with all three, but they recognized his talent both as a pianist and as a composer. He was described as "so stubborn, so bent on having his own way that he had to learn many things by hard experience."[39] Beethoven retained a high regard for Salieri, asking his counsel about composition from time to time and dedicating the set of three violin sonatas, op. 12, to the older composer.

The financial support Beethoven received from Maximillian Franz back in Bonn did not extend beyond early 1794, but the sponsorship of Prince Lichnowsky did much to further his career during his early days in Vienna. Lichnowsky's family and household was a centre of music in Vienna, and Beethoven performed there regularly. At these musical soirées Beethoven also established a reputation for unconventional dress and behaviour. Despite the encouragement and appreciation he received, however, he was a reluctant performer and on occasion had to be enticed into playing by subtle manoeuvres, such as ensuring that the only empty seat left in the room was the stool in front of the piano.[40] Beethoven was highly sensitive and easily provoked to anger, but would subsequently apologize for much more than he was guilty of.[41] The Lichnowsky family put up with his eccentricities because of their early recognition of his enormous talent at the piano.

Wegeler notes Beethoven's "extraordinary" aversion to teaching,[42] but Ferdinand Ries, who became one of Beethoven's pupils, gives a contrary account: "When Beethoven gave me lessons, contrary to his nature, he was extraordinarily patient. I could only attribute this to his love and affection for my father."[43] By 1796, Beethoven was beginning to establish a reputation not only as a performer but also as a composer, with the publication of the set of three piano trios, op. 1, in 1795, and the three piano sonatas, op. 2, the following year. While these early works are structured in the classical tradition of Mozart and Haydn, they also have a distinctive quality. During this time he also developed friendships with other members of the Viennese nobility who were to become his sponsors: Count Andreas Razumovsky, Prince Franz Lobkowitz, Gottfried von Swieten, and later Liechtenstein, Esterhazy, Kinsky, and Archduke Rudolf. Beethoven participated in musical gatherings at their homes and dedicated compositions to one or other of them in recognition of the financial support they provided. In 1796, Beethoven engaged in his first – and as it turned out, his only – concert tour. Over a period of five months he performed in Prague, Berlin, Leipzig, and Dresden. The tour greatly advanced his reputation. The two fine cello sonatas, op. 5, were written at this time and dedicated to Friedrich Wilhelm II of Prussia, for whom Beethoven had given a recital while in Berlin.

Two years later, in 1798, when the French army occupied Vienna, Beethoven met General Bernadotte and conceived the idea of composing a symphony to honour Napoleon.[44] During 1799 and 1800, Beethoven was hard at work on a number of widely acclaimed works, including the Symphony no. 1, op. 21, the Symphony no. 2, op. 36, and the Piano Sonata in C Minor, op. 13 ("Pathétique"). The two symphonies were written in the classical tradition, but the sonata shows the first glimmerings of the "heroic" musical style that became part of Beethoven's second (or middle) period. By 1801, at age thirty, he was becoming conscious of his fame and his unique style, and was able to write the following revealing and confident letter to his friend Franz Wegeler in Bonn: "My compositions bring me in a good deal; and I may say I am offered more commissions than it is possible for me to carry out. Moreover for every composition I can count on six or seven publishers, and even more, if I want them; people no longer come to an arrangement with me, I state my price and they pay. So you can see how pleasantly situated I am."[45] Thayer describes a brief relationship that Beethoven had in 1798 with Magdalena Willmann, a

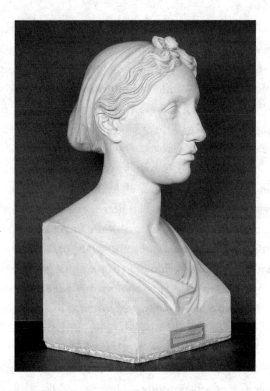

Bust of Giulietta Giucciardi, to whom Beethoven proposed
marriage in 1801, created by Konrad Schweickle (1779–1833).
Beethoven-Haus, Bonn.

young singer in the Vienna State Opera. Beethoven became captivated by her and proposed marriage but she declined, and later married someone else. Thayer asked her niece in 1860 why she had refused Beethoven's advances and her niece is reported to have replied "because he was so ugly and half crazy."[46] In 1800 Beethoven, then aged twenty-nine, met and began giving piano lessons to Guilietta Guicciardi, an attractive aristocratic seventeen-year-old. In November 1801 Beethoven wrote to Franz Wegeler, "But I am leading a slightly more pleasant life – enjoying a few blissful moments ... met a dear charming girl who loves me and whom I love."[47] Beethoven proposed marriage, but her father opposed it on the grounds that Beethoven was "without rank, fortune or permanent engagement." Giulietta eventually married a Count Gallenberg and moved to Italy with him, but she achieved immortality as the dedicatee of the Piano Sonata in C sharp minor, op. 27, no. 2 ("Moonlight"), published in 1801. There is also a sequel to the story of Beethoven's relationship with Giulietta. Twenty-two years later, in a note in French to Anton Schindler (his friend and secretary at the time), he wrote: "I loved her, but not her husband; but she loved him more than me. She told me about his difficulties and gave me 500 Fl. for support. He was always my enemy, which was the reason I tried to do as much good as possible. They married before they went to Italy. She sought me out when crying, but I scorned her ... if I had wished to lose my vital force during my life, what would have been left for those that were noble and better?"[48] The 500 florins were probably in return for the sonata dedication, and his "scorn" likely reflects the difficulty he experienced in coping with emotionality in women. Beethoven seems to be saying that had he married Giulietta, he would not have been able to dedicate his life to his music in the way that he did.

However, a dark cloud was looming on the horizon. In the same letter to Wegeler, only two sentences further on, Beethoven breaks the news about his hearing loss and vividly describes its effects on his music and his lifestyle: "But that jealous demon, my wretched health, has put a nasty spoke in my wheel; and it amounts to this, that for the last three years my hearing has become weaker and weaker." He states that he is constantly afflicted with diarrhea and in consequence suffers from "an extraordinary debility." A physician advised tepid baths in the Danube:

the result was miraculous; my inside improved, but my deafness persisted or became even worse. During this last winter I was truly wretched, for I had really dreadful attacks of colic and again relapsed into my former condition. And thus I remained until about four weeks ago when I went to see (Doctor) Vering. For I began to think that my condition demanded the attention of a surgeon as well; and in any case I had confidence in him. Well, he succeeded in checking almost completely this violent diarrhea. He prescribed tepid baths in the Danube, to which I had always to add a bottle of strengthening ingredients. He ordered no medicines until four days ago when he prescribed pills for my stomach and an infusion for my ear. As a result I have been feeling stronger and better but my ears continue to hum and buzz day and night. I must confess that I lead a miserable life. For almost two years I have ceased to attend any social functions just because I find it impossible to say to people: I am deaf. If I had any other profession I might be able to cope with my infirmity; but in my profession it is a terrible handicap ... in the theatre I have to place myself quite close to the orchestra in order to understand what the actor is saying, and at a distance I cannot hear the high notes of instruments or voices. As for the spoken voice it is surprising that some people have never noticed my deafness; but since I have always been liable to fits of absent-mindedness, they attribute my hardness of hearing to that. Sometimes I can scarcely hear a person who speaks softly; I can hear sounds, it is true, but cannot make out the words. But if anyone shouts I cannot bear it. Heaven only knows what will become of me. Vering [his physician] tells me that my hearing will certainly improve, although my deafness may not be completely cured. Already I have cursed my Creator and my existence. Plutarch has shown me the path of resignation ... Resignation, what a wretched resource! Yet it is all that is left to me.

Beethoven goes on to plead with Wegeler not to tell anyone about his problem.[49]

His friends, however, were not as ignorant as Beethoven had supposed. His pupil Ferdinand Ries recounts a country outing: "I went for a walk in the country with Beethoven and heard a shepherd playing a flute. Beethoven could not hear it and became very quiet and gloomy."[50] In a letter of 1804 to Wegeler, Stephan von Breuning writes: "You cannot conceive, my dear Wegeler, what an indescribable, I might say, fearful effect the gradual loss of hearing has had on him. Think of the feeling of being unhappy in one of such violent temperament; in addition reservedness, mistrust, often toward his best friends, in many things want of decision! ... intercourse with him is a real exertion."[51]

About this time, Beethoven began two other friendships which were to last a lifetime. One was with Karl Amenda (1771–1836), who was born in

Courland in Eastern Poland and had come to Vienna to study music and theology. Music brought them together: Amenda was an accomplished violinist, and they performed together. They had an affectionate relationship as judged by their correspondence and, although Amenda returned to Courland in 1799, he was one of the first to hear about Beethoven's deafness in a letter of 1801.[52] The second friendship was with Nikolaus Zmeskall (1759–1833), who moved to Vienna from Hungary at a young age and spent the rest of his life there. He recognized Beethoven's genius early on, and he became one of his most loyal supporters. The letters that Beethoven wrote to him (about one hundred, which Zmeskall carefully preserved) show that their relationship was casual, close, and unaffected. They often met for meals in one of the taverns in Vienna; he also provided Beethoven with wine and, on occasion, financial help. Beethoven consulted him on domestic problems, particularly his difficulties with servants. Zmeskall developed gout in 1819–20, and so was unable to provide Beethoven with much help toward the end of his life.[53]

Although Beethoven's general health was mostly good during this period, we note the presence of both a long-standing abdominal problem, characterized by colicky pains and diarrhea, and the onset of his hearing loss, which was initially accompanied by extraneous sounds that included humming and buzzing. According to the Fischoff manuscript – a collection of notices and records made by Thayer but derived largely from secondary sources and therefore of doubtful validity – Beethoven had a "dangerous" illness in 1796 or 1797 that settled in his ears and was the cause of his deafness.[54] No details of this illness are available but it has been alleged that it may have been typhus fever or syphilis, both of which can, on occasion, affect the auditory nerve. These conditions and other possible causes for his hearing loss are discussed in chapter 4.

THE HEILIGENSTADT TESTAMENT

Beethoven's distress about his developing deafness led to a serious personal crisis in mid-1802. Professor Schmidt, his physician at the time, recommended that he go to a bathing centre in the country at Heiligenstadt,

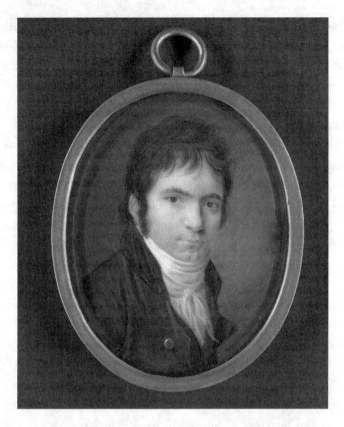

Miniature portrait by Christian Hornemann (1765–1844) of Beethoven at age thirty-two. This painting, done at the time of the Heilegenstadt Testament, captures the composer's focused and expressive features. Collection H.C. Bodmer. Beethoven-Haus, Bonn.

outside of Vienna. Although the setting was delightful, with the fields, flowers and woods that Beethoven so loved, it also was very isolated. During the few months that Beethoven spent there, he reflected on his life, his health (in particular his hearing loss), and his future. In early October that year, he crystallized his thoughts in a document that has come to be known as the Heiligenstadt Testament. This document, written in the

form of a will and dated 6 October 1802, is addressed to his two brothers, Carl and Johann, although Beethoven did not name the latter, likely
because of the conflictual state of their relationship at the time. Once he
had written it, Beethoven likely placed it in a drawer without looking at it
again; it surfaced only six months after his death in 1827. The following
pertinent extracts from this emotional document are very revealing of his
state of mind at the time.[55]

Heiligenstadt, October 6, 1802

For my brothers Carl and .... Beethoven

O my fellow men, who consider me, or describe me as, unfriendly, peevish or
even misanthropic, how greatly do you wrong me. For you do not know the
secret reason why I appear to you to be so. Ever since my childhood my heart
and soul have been imbued with the tender feeling of goodwill; and I have always
been ready to perform even great actions. But just think, for the last six years I
have been afflicted with an incurable complaint which has been made worse by
incompetent doctors. From year to year my hopes of being cured have gradually
been shattered and finally I have been forced to accept the prospect of a <u>perma-
nent infirmity</u> (the curing of which may perhaps take years or may even prove
to be impossible). Though endowed with a passionate and lively temperament
and even fond of the distractions offered by society I was soon obliged to seclude
myself and live in solitude. If at times I decided just to ignore my infirmity, alas!,
how cruelly was I then driven back by the intensified sad experience of my poor
hearing. Yet I could not bring myself to say to people: "Speak up, shout, for I am
deaf." Alas! How could I possibly refer to the impairing of one sense which in me
should be more perfectly developed than in other people, a sense which at one
time I possessed in the greatest perfection, even to a degree of perfection such
as assuredly few in my profession possess or have ever possessed – Oh, I cannot
do it; so forgive me, if you ever see me withdrawing from your company which
I used to enjoy. Moreover my misfortune pains me doubly, inasmuch as it leads
to my being misunderstood. For me there can be no relaxation in human society,
no refined conversations, no mutual confidences. I must live quite alone and may
creep into society only as often as sheer necessity demands; I must live like an
outcast. If I appear in company I am overcome by a burning anxiety, a fear that

I am running the risk of letting people notice my condition – And that has been my experience during the last six months which I have spent in the country. My sensible doctor by suggesting that I should spare my hearing as much as possible has more or less encouraged my present natural inclination, though indeed when carried away now and then by my instinctive desire for human society, I have let myself be tempted to seek it. But how humiliated I have felt if somebody standing beside me heard the sound of a flute in the distance and <u>I heard nothing</u>, or if somebody heard <u>a shepherd sing and</u> again I heard nothing – Such experiences almost made me despair, and I was on the point of putting an end to my life – The only thing that held me back was my art. For indeed it seemed to be impossible to leave this world before I had produced all the works that I felt the urge to compose; and thus I have dragged on this miserable existence – a truly miserable existence, seeing that I have such a sensitive body that any fairly sudden change can plunge me from the best spirits into the worst of humors ... And you, my brothers Carl and .... when I am dead, request on my behalf Professor Schmidt, if he is still living, to describe my disease, and attach this written document to his record, so that after my death at any rate the world and I may be reconciled as far as possible ... It was thanks to virtue and also to my art that I did not put an end to my life by suicide ... Joyfully I go to meet Death – should it come before I have had an opportunity of developing all my artistic gifts, then in spite of my hard fate it would still come too soon, and no doubt I would like it to postpone its coming – Yet even so I should be content, for would it not free me from a condition of continual suffering? Come then, Death, <u>whenever</u> you like, and with courage I will go to meet you – Farewell; and when I am dead, do not wholly forget me. I deserve to be remembered by you, since during my lifetime I have often thought of you and tried to make you happy – Be happy –
Ludwig van Beethoven

From this document, it is not difficult to see that Beethoven was going through a mental depression. He describes severe distress because of his increasing deafness and the realization that this likely would be permanent; he is irritable or "peevish" and "misanthropic"; he is suspicious to the point of feeling he is being shunned as an outcast by society; he is preoccupied with death and even reveals that it is only his virtue and his art that have prevented him from committing suicide. The Heiligenstadt Testament is a *cri de coeur* from the depths of his being, representing a crisis and a turning point in Beethoven's career. Marek calls it "one of the most heartbreaking documents to be found in the long literature of lamentations." Beethoven's awareness of his deafness and the perception of the impact that this would have on his musical career, was a key issue. With the courage of genius he turned his crisis into an opportunity and a challenge. His increasing subsequent focus on composing, rather than conducting or performing and the fact that from then on he referred to his hearing loss only infrequently in his letters indicates that he found a way of coping with his impairment. He immersed himself in his music, and above all in composition. It is during this period that his music changed from the "classical" style of the first period to the "heroic" style of his second.

THE SECOND VIENNA (HEROIC) PERIOD

The years between 1802 and 1812 were the most productive of Beethoven's career: compositions include six symphonies (nos. 3 to 8), two piano concertos (nos. 4 and 5), an opera (*Fidelio*), a violin concerto, five string quartets (nos. 7 to 11), and seven piano sonatas. The style of his second period is not only "heroic" but also expansive, in particular an expansion of form. This music expresses a wide range of moods, from the drama and excitement of *Fidelio* to the congenial dialogue of Piano Sonata in E minor, op. 90; from the intensity and fateful symbolism of the Symphony no. 5 to the joy and serenity of the Symphony no. 6 ("Pastoral"). Many of Beethoven's contemporaries had difficulty in adjusting to these changes in style from the familiar harmonies of the classical period, even though the changes are more structural than harmonic. Those people he called his enemies. Nevertheless, his works were widely played and appreciated. The quality and the theory of these developments in musical style are well described by William Kinderman and Donald Francis Tovey.[56]

Beethoven's relationships with three women – Eleonore von Breuning, Magdalena Willmann, and Giulietta Giucciardi – were described above.

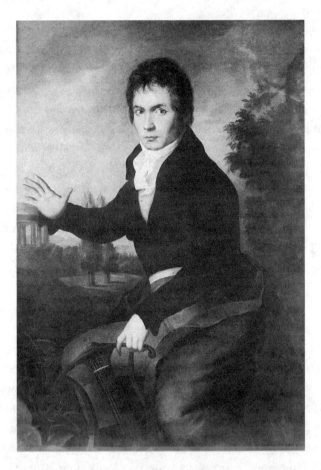

*Reproduction of a Romantic full-length painting by Willibrord
Joseph Mähler (1778–1860) of Beethoven in 1804, during the early
part of his second Vienna period. Beethoven-Haus, Bonn.*

His remaining relationships all occurred during this second period,
although that with Countess Marie Erdödy extended well into the third
period. Beethoven's relationships with women have been a topic of endless fascination and controversy among scholars. He certainly fell in love
on a number of occasions during his lifetime and even proposed marriage to at least three women, but he never married. There has been much

speculation but no certainty on the question as to whether he ever lost his virginity. Thayer refers to a prayer written by Beethoven in 1817, part of which suggests some experience of sexuality: "Sensual enjoyment without a union of souls is bestial and will always remain bestial; after it one experiences not a trace of a noble sentiment but rather regret."[57] However, the bestial analogy can also be interpreted as Beethoven's justification for not seeking out non-loving sexual relationships.[58]

In appearance, Beethoven had a short and stocky build with long and untidy hair. His height was about 167 centimetres and his face was marked with circular scars, the result either of smallpox during his childhood or severe acne during his teens. His clothes were generally clean but untidy. When he walked he leaned his whole body forward, but he was not bent. Stephan von Breuning explained that in a curious way he was attractive to women despite not being handsome.[59] In social settings he seems to have had a commanding presence. Schlosser, whose biography of Beethoven was published in 1827,[60] gives the following description: "To every human being it was immediately apparent that Beethoven was a remarkable human being. His walk was animated, his mouth was expressive, and his eyes betrayed the enormous depth of his feeling. But it was his magnificent forehead that revealed his majestic creative force. When he displayed a friendly mien, it had the charm of childlike innocence; when he smiled one believed not only in him but in all of mankind. At such times his every word, motion and glance seemed sincere and genuine."[61]

Accounts of Beethoven's relationships with women written by his friends have only served to obscure the issue because of their disagreement. Wegeler wrote, "The truth is that Beethoven was never not in love and was usually involved to a high degree," and, "In Vienna Beethoven was always involved in a love affair and sometimes made conquests which would have been difficult if not impossible for many an Adonis."[62] Ries states that Beethoven enjoyed looking at women and that lovely, youthful faces particularly pleased him. He describes an evening when he went to visit Beethoven and found him sitting on the sofa with a handsome young woman. He made to leave, but Beethoven asked Ries to play romantic pieces on the piano, which he did. The woman subsequently left, and Beethoven and Ries followed her for a while, Beethoven stating that he did not know her. Ries later found out that she was the mistress of a foreign prince.[63] This is a curious anecdote: Ries seems to be saying that Beethoven was entertaining a woman he did not know, and that he requested romantic music rather than privacy, and he gives no explanation as to why the woman left or why they followed her. Anton Schindler, who was Beethoven's secretary in the last few years of his life gives a different picture but does not clarify the details. Schindler believed that Beethoven was morally chaste throughout his life, and that he was as "upright as Cato" in the matter of morality, but he conceded that Beethoven's reputation as a "woman hater" grew after he won the custody battle for Karl.[64] Schindler states that Beethoven's various love affairs must be treated with discretion and he chides those "French and German writers" who were more interested in Beethoven's love life than in his music.[65] Schindler also refers to Madame Cherubini, who told Beethoven that the reason he found so little satisfaction in his relationships with women was that he was too "brusque," and his ideals were too high.[66]

One of these thwarted relationships was with Josephine von Brunswick. The Brunswick family were aristocratic landowners from Hungary who had moved to Vienna in 1799 after the death of their father, the Count. The family consisted of a son, Franz, and three daughters, Therese, Josephine, and Charlotte, who were respectively five, nine, and twelve years younger than Beethoven. He gave piano lessons to the three girls, and subsequently developed lasting friendships with Franz and Therese, both of whom were talented musicians; Therese was also an artist. Shortly after the family's arrival in Vienna, a marriage was arranged between Josephine, who was then twenty, and a Count Joseph Deym, aged forty-seven. She married against her wishes in order to oblige her mother, and they had three children in less than four years. The count died from tuberculosis early in 1804, while she was pregnant with their fourth child. When Beethoven renewed his friendship with Josephine and started giving her piano lessons again, their relationship intensified. This caused considerable distress to her sisters, who attempted to discourage the relationship. There are six extant letters from Beethoven to Josephine written in the

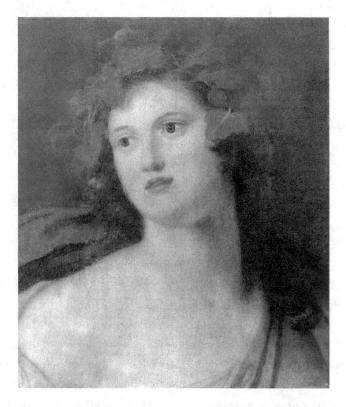

Portrait of Josephine Deym (née von Brunswick) by Johann Lampi
(1751–1830). Josephine had piano lessons from Beethoven in 1799, when
she was twenty, and in 1804, after the death of her husband. Beethoven wrote six
passionate letters to her in 1805 but although she liked and admired him,
she rejected his advances. Beethoven-Haus, Bonn.

second half of 1805, and several of her replies.[67] Beethoven expresses his feelings with passion, but Beethoven's fervent expressions of love went unrequited, as is apparent from the following extracts:

Oh, beloved Josephine, it is no desire for the other sex that draws me to you, no, it is just you, your whole self with all your individual qualities ... you have conquered me ... Oh you, you make me hope that your heart will long – beat for me – Mine can only – cease – to beat for you – when – it no longer beats.[68]

There is no language which can express what is far above all mere regard ... only in music – Alas, am I not too proud when I believe that music is more at my command than words ... You, you, my all, my happiness – even in my music I cannot do so.[69]

I love you as dearly as you do not love me.[70]

Am I really unable to influence you? – although you have so great an influence on me – and make me so happy.[71]

In one of her letters, she replies: "You have long had my heart, dear Beethoven ... The possession of my noblest self. Do not tear my heart apart – do not try to persuade me further. I love you inexpressibly, as one gentle soul does another. Are you not capable of this covenant? I am not receptive to other forms of love for the present."[72] In a subsequent letter she wrote, "Even before I knew you, your music made me enthusiastic for you – the goodness of your character, your affection increased it. This preference that you granted me would have been the finest jewel of my life if you had loved me less sensually. That I cannot satisfy this sensual love makes you angry with me, but I would have to violate holy bonds if I gave heed to your longings."[73]

Although she was a widow, and therefore free to marry if she so desired, Josephine rejected Beethoven's advances. According to her sister Therese's memoirs, published many years later, Josephine had refused him because of "mother-love for her four young children," and because "he lacked a woman because he did not know how to act." However, Therese also reproached herself for having contributed to the breakup of the relationship between Josephine and Beethoven. In 1848, twenty-one years after Beethoven's death, she wrote in her journal, "Beethoven was intimately linked in spirit with Josephine ... they were born for each other ... they would both still be alive if they had come together."[74]

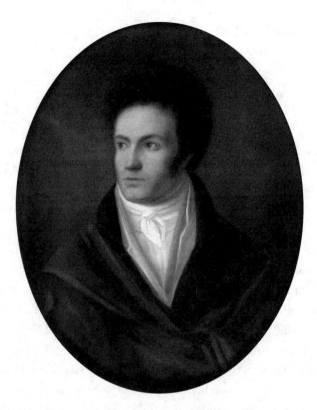

Half-length painting by Isadore Neugass (ca 1780–ca 1847)
of Beethoven in 1806, at the height of his second Vienna period.
Beethoven-Haus, Bonn.

In five further extant letters to Josephine, all written in 1807,[75] Beethoven is friendly and affectionate but more formal. In the last of these letters he seems to have reluctantly come to terms with her decision to rebuff him: "I thank you for wishing still to appear as if I were not altogether banished from your memory, even though this came about perhaps more at the instigation of others."

In 1807, Beethoven had a brief and curious relationship with Marie Bigot, a woman from Colmar in Alsace, France, who had come to Vienna

with her husband, a librarian. Bigot was an excellent pianist and performed both Haydn's and Beethoven's music in public. Beethoven became
enthralled with both her and her interpretation of his music. On 4 March
1807 he wrote, addressing her as "My dear and much admired Marie!"
inviting her and her infant daughter, but specifically not her husband
because he "presumably has gone out already," for a drive in the country
for "the delightful enjoyment of Nature's glorious beauties," adding, "It
would be quite alien to the outlook of our so enlightened and cultured
Marie if for the sake of mere scruples she were to rob me of my greatest
pleasure – Oh, whatever reasons you may put forward for not accepting
my proposal, I shall ascribe your refusal to nothing else but to distrust of
my character – and I shall never believe that you cherish sincere friendship for me … Now, send me a reply, dear M., whether you can come – I
am not asking you whether you want to come – for I should interpret the
latter only to my disadvantage."[76] Unfortunately for Beethoven, Marie
refused the invitation and also told her husband, who must have expressed
dismay at Beethoven's initiative; on the following day Beethoven wrote
two extended letters, the first to M. Bigot and the second to the couple.[77]
In both letters he expresses his fondness for the couple, denies that he had
any motive other than friendship: "I did so merely in order to induce you
to enjoy the beautiful fine day. I was thinking far more of your pleasure
than my own … never, never will you find me dishonourable." The style,
repetition, and extensive detail of these two letters clearly indicate that a
defensive Beethoven was "protesting too much," and that there was likely
an ulterior motive to his invitation. Nothing is known of any further relationship or correspondence with Marie, although Beethoven wrote four
further business letters to M. Bigot in 1807 and 1808. In 1809 the couple
returned to France, where Marie became a well-known teacher, counting
the young Felix Mendelssohn among her pupils. Georgette Jeanclaude
wrote a charming historical novel about the relationship between Marie
Bigot and Beethoven.[78]

Beethoven had an extended relationship with Anna Marie Erdödy, a
countess who, originally from Hungary, had separated from her husband
and was living in Vienna with her three children. Erdödy was a pianist

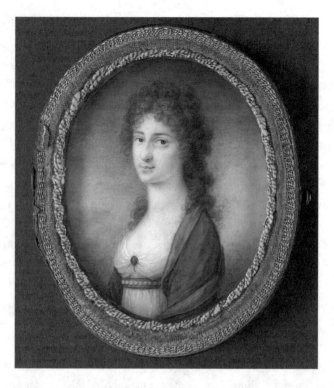

Portrait of Anna Maria Erdödy with whom Beethoven had an
extended but likely platonic relationship between 1807 and 1822.
Artist unknown. Beethoven-Haus, Bonn.

and was highly appreciative of Beethoven's music. It is uncertain how they met, but for a few months in late 1807 and 1808, Beethoven rented an apartment in her home, together with other tenants. In his first extant letter to the Countess, from March 1809, Beethoven asks her forgiveness for having acted wrongly, but provides no detail of the event.[79] Over the next ten years there are eleven further letters from Beethoven to the Countess, with a four-year gap between May 1811 and February 1815. The style and content of these letters is friendly and businesslike; though affectionate, they do not have the quality of love letters. Some are replies to her

letters; unfortunately none of her letters have survived, although we do
have two brief poems that she wrote him: "I've come from Jedlesee as mes-
senger / To him who next to God is the greatest composer," and "Thou
greatest of the great spirits / Supreme master of music / Whom all Europe
now knows / Hear our prayer, Remain in our midst."[80] In October 1815,
Erdödy left Austria, never to return. The following May, Beethoven wrote
a supportive letter of condolence to her on the death of her son.[81] She had
been through great personal and family difficulties, and Beethoven con-
soles her: "We finite beings, who are the embodiment of an infinite spirit,
are born to suffer both pain and joy; and one might almost say that the
best of us obtain joy through suffering."[82] In June 1817 Beethoven wrote to
her from Heiligenstadt; this letter includes a number of details about his
medical problems, his doctor, and the treatments he was undergoing,

My beloved suffering Friend, My dearest Countess! Of late I have been tossed
about far too much and overwhelmed with too many cares. Then after feeling
constantly unwell since October 6th 1816 I developed on October 15th a violent
feverish cold, so that I had to stay in bed for a very long time; and only after
several months was I allowed to go out even for a short while. Until now the after
effects of this illness could not be dispelled. I changed my doctors, because my
own doctor, a wily Italian, [Dr Malfatti] had powerful secondary motives where
I was concerned and lacked both honesty and intelligence. That was in April
1817. Well, from April 15th until May 4th I had to take six powders daily and
six bowls of tea. That treatment lasted until May 4th. After that I had to take
another kind of powder, also six times daily; and I had to rub myself three times
a day with a volatile ointment. Then I had to come here where I am taking baths.
Since yesterday I have been taking another medicine, namely a tincture, of which
I have to swallow 12 spoonfuls daily – Every day I hope to see the end of this
distressing condition. Although my health has improved a little, yet it will be a
long time apparently before I am completely cured. You can imagine how all this
must affect the rest of my existence. My hearing has become worse; and as I have
never been able to look after myself and my needs, I am even less able to do so
now; and my cares have been increased still further by the responsibility for my
brother's child.[83]

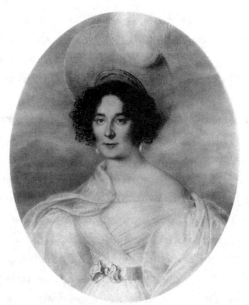

Portrait of Therese Malfatti, the niece of Beethoven's physician
Giovanni Malfatti. Beethoven had a brief relationship with her in 1810,
when she was eighteen, and proposed marriage, but she
rebuffed him, likely on the advice of her father.
Artist unknown. Beethoven-Haus, Bonn.

There is no evidence, either in Beethoven's letters to Countess Erdödy or in any other sources, to suggest that their relationship was anything more than a close friendship of kindred spirits. In the early stages it may have been primarily a business relationship involving her financial support in return for dedication of music to her; later on, their friendship was likely based on mutual support and affection during the personal, family, and health problems they were both experiencing.

In 1810, Beethoven had a brief relationship with Therese Malfatti, the seventeen-year-old niece of his current physician, Dr Giovanni Malfatti. The one extant letter from Beethoven to Therese is dated May 1810. In it, he expresses his affection for her, encloses her a composition (likely *Für Elise*, WoO59), and hopes to "ramble for a while through bushes, woods, under trees, through grass and around rocks. No one can love the country as much as I do. For surely woods, trees and rocks produce the echo which man desires to hear."[84]

Around this time Beethoven became concerned about his personal appearance: he asked friends to purchase mirrors and neck cloths for him, and even visited a tailor to purchase some suits. He also wrote to his friend Franz Wegeler, who lived at Coblenz, not far from his birthplace at Bonn, asking him to obtain a copy of his baptismal certificate, with careful instructions not to confuse him with his brother Ludwig Maria, who had been born and died before Beethoven's birth.[85] It was likely only then, on receiving the certificate, that Beethoven learned he had been born in 1770 and was thus forty rather than thirty-eight years old. Because of these events, it is thought that Beethoven proposed marriage to Therese but was rebuffed (probably by her father, rather than by Therese herself); a mutual friend of both Beethoven and Therese conveyed this information to Beethoven, who responded: "Your news has again plunged me from the heights of the sublime ecstasy down into the depths."[86] Beethoven had friendly relationships with a number of other women in his lifetime, including Bettina Brentano and Amalie Sebald, but there is little evidence of a deeper emotional involvement. In 1817, he had a brief, transient relationship with a married woman known only as "T," but very little is known about this.[87]

One of the most important relationships, however, was with a woman who has come to be known as the "Immortal Beloved."[88] After Beethoven's death in 1827, his friends found three letters in a locked drawer in his apartment, all written during a two-day period, 6 and 7 July, with no year and no named addressee. Because these letters reveal so much about Beethoven's feelings for the woman, the complete text of all three is given below:[89]

[Teplitz, July 6 and 7, 1812]
July 6th, in the morning

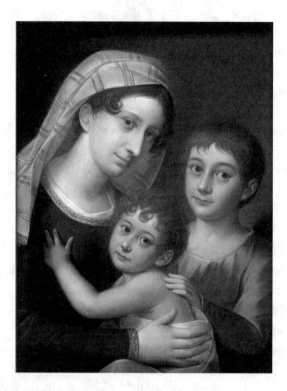

Antonie Brentano, who lived in Vienna from 1809 to 1812, is
probably the intended recipient of Beethoven's letters written in 1812
to an "unknown beloved." This portrait by Nikolaus Lauer (fl 1794–1804)
shows her with Georg and Fanny, two of her children.
Beethoven-Haus, Bonn.

My angel, my all, my very self. – Only a few words today, and, what is more, written in pencil (and with your pencil) – I shan't be certain of my rooms here until
tomorrow; what an unnecessary waste of time is all this – Why this profound
sorrow, when necessity speaks – can our love endure without sacrifices, without
our demanding everything from one another; can you alter the fact that you are
not wholly mine, that I am not wholly yours? – Dear God, look at Nature in all
her beauty and set your heart at rest about what must be – Love demands all,

and rightly so, and thus it is for me with you, for you with me – But you forget so easily that I must live for me and for you; if we were completely united, you would feel this painful necessity just as little as I do – My journey was dreadful and I did not arrive here until yesterday at four o'clock in the morning. As there were few horses the mail coach chose another route, but what a dreadful road it was; at the last stage but one I was warned not to travel by night; attempts were made to frighten me about a forest, but all this only spurred me on to proceed – and it was wrong of me to do so. The coach broke down, of course, owing to the dreadful road which had not been made up was nothing but a country track. If I hadn't had those two postilions I should have been left stranded on the way – On the other ordinary road Esterhazy with eight horses met with the same fate as I did with four – Yet I felt to a certain extent the pleasure I always feel when I have overcome some difficulty successfully – Well, let me turn quickly from outer to inner experiences. No doubt we shall meet soon; and today also time fails me to tell you of the thoughts which during these last few days I have been revolving about my life – If our hearts were always closely united, I would certainly entertain no such thoughts. My heart overflows with a longing to tell you so many things – Oh – there are moments when I find that speech is quite inadequate – Be cheerful – and be for ever my faithful, my only sweetheart, my all, as I am yours. The gods must send us everything else, whatever must and shall be our fate – Your faithful Ludwig

Monday evening, July 6th
You are suffering, you, my most precious one – I have noticed this very moment that letters have to be handed in very early, on Monday – or on Thursday – the only days when the mail coach goes from here to K. – You are suffering – Oh, where I am, you are with me – I will see to it that you and I, that I can live with you. What life!!!!! as it is now !!!! without you – pursued by the kindness of people here and there, a kindness that I think – that I wish to deserve just as little as I deserve it – man's homage to man – that pains me – and when I consider myself in the setting of the universe, what am I and what is that man – whom one calls the greatest of men – and yet – on the other hand therein lies the divine element of man – I weep when I think that probably you will not receive the first news of me until Saturday – However much you love me – my love for you is even greater

– but never conceal yourself from me – good night – Since I am taking the baths I must get off to sleep – Dear God – so near! So far! Is not our love truly founded in heaven – and, what is as strongly cemented as the firmament of Heaven? –

Good morning, on July 7th

Even when I am in bed my thoughts rush to you, my eternally beloved, now and then joyfully, then again sadly, waiting to know whether Fate will hear our prayer – To face life I must live altogether with you or never see you. Yes, I am resolved to be a wanderer abroad until I can fly to your arms and say that I have found my true home with you and enfolded in your arms can let my soul be wafted to the realm of blessed spirits – alas unfortunately it must be so – You will become composed, the more so as you know that I am faithful to you; no other woman can ever possess my heart – never – never – Oh God, why must one be separated from her who is so dear. Yet my life in V[ienna] at present is a miserable life – Your love has made me both the happiest and the unhappiest of mortals – At my age I now need stability and regularity in my life – can this coexist with our relationship? – Angel, I have just heard that the post goes every day – and therefore I must close, so that you may receive the letter immediately – Be calm; for only by calmly considering our lives can we achieve our purpose to live together – Be calm – love me – Today – yesterday – what tearful longing for you – for you – you – my life – my all – all good wishes to you – Oh, do continue to love me – never misjudge your lover's most faithful heart. ever yours – ever mine – L – ever ours.

These letters have aroused intense interest among biographers who for one hundred and fifty years have had a field day speculating about who the recipient might have been. Marek suggests seven possible recipients, and lists the biographers favouring each one, but concludes that the woman's true identity was Dorothea Ertmann.[90] In a detailed analysis of the letter, and of Beethoven's various relationships, Rolland concludes that the recipient was Therese von Brunswick.[91] Schindler identified Giulietta Guiccardi.[92] Thayer, after considering all the possibilities, does not commit himself. From the text of the letters it is clear that Beethoven had passionate feelings toward the recipient and that he wished, although not too hopefully, that the relationship would continue. It is also clear that his feelings were reciprocated. A further question arises as to whether the letters were ever sent, and if they were, whether Beethoven kept a copy, or whether the recipient returned originals. We will likely never know for sure, but this has not stopped speculations.

Maynard Solomon carried out a meticulous analysis of the letters, their context, and the recent travels of both Beethoven and all possible recipients.[93] The three letters were written shortly after Beethoven arrived at Teplitz at the end of a journey from Vienna via Prague, and it seems he met the recipient while passing through Prague. Solomon traces the movements of all the women Beethoven knew during that key period, and concludes that the "Immortal Beloved" was almost certainly Antonie Brentano, the wife of Franz Brentano. Most scholars who have discussed this topic since then appear to agree with Solomon. Although Marek – who was writing before Solomon published his monograph naming Antonie – did consider her as a possible recipient, he concludes she is not a candidate because she was happily married to Franz: "The evidence of their relationship is clear and excludes even a remote chance of anything but friendship ... in none of [the letters from Beethoven to the Brentanos] is there the slightest sign of a romantic involvement with Antonie."[94] Rolland also considered and ruled out Antonie Brentano on the basis that Beethoven's friendship with Antonie and Franz Brentano was "marked by respect, and was also a little distant."[95]

Antonie and Franz Brentano lived in Vienna from 1809 to 1812 and had become friends with Beethoven particularly because of their appreciation for his music. In November 1812 they moved to Frankfurt, where Franz remained as a businessman, and they never returned to Vienna. Beethoven wrote several letters to each of them after their departure from Vienna: to Antonie, one letter in 1815 and three in 1816; to Franz, one each in 1816 and 1817, two in 1821, three in 1822, and one in 1823. In his letter to Antonie of February 1816, Beethoven encloses a copper engraving on which his face is stamped taken from the Brentano portrait.[96] The later letters to Franz deal largely with business: Franz had lent Beethoven some money and Beethoven made arrangements to repay the loan, and Franz also acted as Beethoven's agent in his (sometimes tortuous) negotiations with pub-

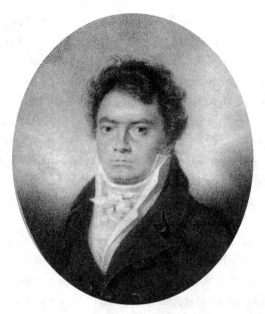

Painting of Beethoven by Blassius Höfel (1792–1863), based on a
pencil drawing by Louis Latronne (1790–1842), and printed in Vienna
by Artaria and Col. in 1814. It is likely that Beethoven sent the original
copper engraving of this portrait, painted in 1814, to Antonie Brentano,
saying "several people maintain that in this picture they can discern my
soul quite clearly but I offer no opinion on that point" (Emily Anderson, ed.
and trans. Letters of Beethoven, *2: 557–8). Ira F. Brilliant Center for*
Beethoven Studies, San José State University, CA.

lishers. The letters to both Antonie and Franz are warm and friendly; the
engraving is the only hint of an emotional involvement with Antonie, and
in his letters to Franz there is no suggestion of anxiety, guilt, or defensive-
ness that might indicate a sexual relationship with Franz's wife.

In February 1819 Antonie wrote a remarkable letter to J.M. Sailer.[97]
Sailer was an orator, educator, and priest who ran Landshut University
in Bavaria. At the height of his custody dispute with Johanna over Karl,

Beethoven secured the help of Antonie, who wrote to Sailer supporting Karl's admission "to a Catholic University that is not too expensive." She displays great affection for Beethoven and strongly takes his side in the custody battle. She concludes her letter by stating: "This great, excellent man … is even greater as a human being than as an artist … he is natural, simple, and wise, with pure intentions," and she signs herself "Winkler Hausfrau" (housewife from Winkler). This letter, dated seven years after the "Immortal Beloved" messages, indicates that she still had strong feelings of affection for Beethoven, stating that he is "even greater as a human being than an artist," a great compliment. It seems clear that Beethoven did fall in love with Antonie, that he saw her in Prague on his way to Teplitz from Vienna in the summer of 1812, and that he addressed the three famous letters after their meeting. It is also probable that the letters were never sent. Beethoven did not make nor keep copies of his letters, and it is even less likely that Antonie received the letters and then returned them. Beethoven knew the relationship had no future, partly because of his own ambivalence about commitment and sexuality, partly because of her marital status and membership in the aristocracy. In writing the letters, he satisfied his feelings of affection in his imagination and was able to experience his passion vicariously; the act of writing may perhaps also have enabled him obtain a form of closure to a relationship that he knew was terminating.

Lund alleges that Beethoven was the father of Antonie's son Karl Josef, who was born on 8 March 1813, eight months after the letters were written[98] but while she pulls together much circumstantial evidence, the argument is diminished by overstating the case. She also speculates that both Schindler and Thayer knew Antonie Brentano was the "Immortal Beloved" but had attempted a "cover up" by pointing the finger at other candidates. It seems unlikely that the relationship was ever consummated. The letter contain no references to the recipient's physical appearance or beauty, which might be expected if there had been a sexual dimension to their relationship. Antonie's references to Beethoven's "greatness as a human being" and his "pure intentions" in her letter to Sailer also support this conclusion. It is also probable that Beethoven's feelings for Antonie extended late into his life, as he dedicated the Diabelli Variations, op. 120, published in 1823, to her, and the Piano Sonata in E major, op. 109, to Antonie's daughter Maximiliana; he also intended to dedicate the next two piano sonatas, op. 110 and 111, to Antonie, but in the end did not do so.[99] These final piano works are filled with beauty and passion and are among Beethoven's greatest compositions.

Although Beethoven never saw Antonie after their departure from Vienna, it is clear that they retained a deep mutual respect and affection for each other. There appears to have been no falling out, as happened frequently to Beethoven's relationships, and her feelings for him appear genuine and enduring. We cannot know why the Brentanos left Vienna for Frankfurt, but since they left within a few months of the "Immortal Beloved" letters, one cannot help wondering if the departure may not have been precipitated by the relationship, to help Antonie overcome her attachment to Beethoven and restore her relationship with her husband. Antonie lived a long life (she died in 1869 at age eighty-nine, surviving her husband by twenty-five years) but she never revealed a deeper relationship with Beethoven. Yet until she died she retained several artefacts and memorabilia sent to her by a mutual friend after Beethoven's death.[100]

There is one further possible reference to Antonie as the "A" in a prayer Beethoven wrote at the end of 1812 (six months after the letters, around the time of the Brentano's departure from Vienna): "Submission, absolute submission to your fate – only this can give you the sacrifice … Thou mayest no longer be a man, not for thyself, only for others, for thee there is no longer happiness except in thyself, in thy art – O God give me strength to conquer myself, nothing must chain me to life. Thus everything connected with A will go to destruction."[101] If "A" indeed refers to Antonie, as appears probable given the timing and the context, this prayer represents another *cri de coeur* in which Beethoven implores divine intervention to help him accept the permanent end to their relationship. His emphatic statement that he "may no longer be a man" indicates his awareness that this was likely his last opportunity to have a lasting and loving relationship. He seems also to be making a choice between his art and his relationship with "A," and that his art will only flourish if "everything con-

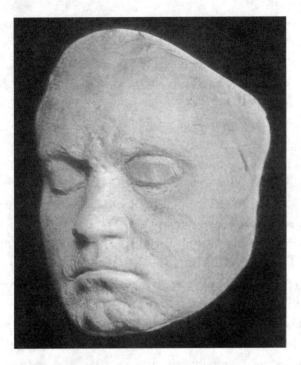

Life mask of Beethoven created by Franz Klein (1779–1840)
in 1812, the year of Beethoven's letters to an "unknown beloved"
and his meeting with Goethe. Beethoven-Haus, Bonn.

nected with A" is destroyed. We can only speculate on what might have
happened had he indeed chosen Antonie over his music.

Mention must be made about the relationship between Beethoven and
Goethe, Germany's two leading men of arts during this period. Goethe's
key role in bridging the German Enlightenment of the eighteenth century
with the Romantic movement of the nineteenth was discussed in chapter
1. Goethe and Beethoven had admired each other from afar for some years,
and Bettina Brentano (Franz Brentano's half-sister) arranged a meeting
between them at Teplitz in the summer of 1812.[102] Unlike Beethoven,
Goethe had an aristocratic background and bearing, and at the time of

their meeting likely had an even wider reputation than did Beethoven. The meeting went well at a superficial level, but Goethe made some gently critical comments about Beethoven to friends after their parting.[103] In a letter to Zelter, for example, Goethe wrote "Unfortunately, he is an utterly untamed personality, not at all in the wrong if he finds the world detestable, but he thereby does not make it more enjoyable either for himself or for others. He is very much to be excused, on the other hand, and very much to be pitied, as his hearing is leaving him, which, perhaps, injures the musical part of his nature less than the social. He, by nature laconic, becomes more so because of this lack." A possibly apocryphal anecdote has been told of the two walking together through Teplitz: Goethe expressed his annoyance at the constant respectful greetings of passersby and Beethoven responded, "Do not let that trouble your Excellency, perhaps the greetings are intended for me."[104] (Perhaps history has borne out Beethoven's rather arrogant reply, in that he is now the more widely recognized of the two.) Rolland and others have written extensively about this meeting and about the relationship between these two great German artists.[105]

During this period, Beethoven was also involved with his brother Johann, who had moved to Vienna in 1793 shortly after Beethoven and found a job in an apothecary shop. Johann worked hard, saved carefully, and within a few years was able to purchase his own business as an apothecary. In a letter to Johann in 1796, while he was away on a concert tour, Beethoven writes: "I hope that you will enjoy living in Vienna more and more, but do be on your guard against the whole tribe of bad women."[106] Johann's apothecary's business prospered, and in 1809 he made a considerable profit by providing the French army with drugs during their occupation of Linz, where he lived at the time.[107] By 1819, he had purchased a large country estate at Gneixendorf, about sixty kilometres from Vienna. From time to time he lent money to Beethoven, which placed a strain on their relationship. A minor crisis between them occurred in 1812, when Johann, still a bachelor at thirty-five, took in a housekeeper named Therese, who then became his mistress. Ludwig traveled to Linz, determined to break up the relationship, and appealed to both the bishop and the police for help, but Johann, increasingly angered by his brother's interference in his private affairs, played his trump card by marrying Therese.[108] Subsequently Johann played little part in Beethoven's affairs until the final years of the composer's life.

These difficulties likely had some impact on Beethoven's health, although the period from 1805 to 1810 contains relatively few health references. He continued to experience episodes of abdominal pain: in a letter of 1805 he refers to this pain briefly, stating that he cannot come to a rehearsal of his opera (*Fidelio*) because "since yesterday I have been suffering from colic pains – my usual complaint."[109] In 1808, he refers to "wretched attacks of colic" that interfere with his activities,[110] and in a letter of 1810 to his close friend Nikolaus Zmeskall he describes "another violent attack of colic."[111]

Beethoven refers to depression on two occasions. The first is in a letter to Franz Wegeler in Bonn asking Wegeler to send a copy of his baptismal certificate;[112] he gives no reason for the request, but at the time he was courting and hoping to marry Therese Malfatti. In this letter he states, "But who can escape the onslaughts of tempests raging around him? Yet I should be happy, perhaps one of the happiest of mortals, if that fiend had not settled in my ears – If I had not read somewhere that a man should not voluntarily quit this life so long as he can still perform a good deed, I would have left this earth long ago – and, what is more, by my own hand – Oh, this life is indeed beautiful, but for me it is poisoned forever." The second reference to depression comes in December 1813 in a letter to a lawyer in Prague,[113] in which he writes: "In everything I undertake in Vienna I am surrounded by innumerable enemies. I am on the verge of despair. My brother [most likely Carl] ... is – my greatest enemy." This statement indicates not only depression but also possible paranoid ideas. Beethoven had a complex relationship with his brother Carl, especially after the latter's marriage in 1806. Times of affection and devotion were punctuated by episodes of intense conflict and animosity when the brothers even came to blows – as happened in 1813 around the time the above letter was written.[114] Much of this conflict revolved around money: it seems that Carl had even more difficulty than Beethoven in managing his finances.

Beethoven's lifelong anxiety about money became more severe as he grew older. He was almost wholly dependent on compositions for his income, particularly as his deafness increased to the point that he could no longer perform, teach, or conduct. At certain periods through his life he had the benefit of regular stipends from aristocratic or affluent sponsors, but even with lifetime guarantees, circumstances changed and the income was reduced or stopped altogether. For example, in 1809 he received an invitation from the King of Westphalia to perform there periodically, in exchange for a salary of 600 gold ducats for life and 150 ducats traveling expenses,[115] but this agreement never materialized, likely because Beethoven felt constrained by the requirement to travel to Westphalia. A group of three Viennese gentlemen – Archduke Rudolf, Prince Lobkowitz, and Prince Kinsky – set up an arrangement with Beethoven whereby they would provide him with an annual salary of 5,000 florins on condition that he remain in Vienna, and an agreement was signed by all parties. This arrangement worked for only two years. By 1811 the war with France had strained Austria's finances to such an extent that the state treasury was bankrupt, and severe inflation set in. As a result Prince Lobkowitz could no longer maintain his contributions. Then, in November 1812 Prince Kinsky was killed in a fall from his horse; the resulting costly and protracted legal wrangles with the heirs to Kinsky's estate were only resolved by compromise in 1815.[116]

Archduke Rudolf (1788–1831), the third signatory of Beethoven's pension agreement, also became a lifelong pupil, sponsor, friend, and admirer. He was a nephew of Emperor Joseph II and apparently suffered from epilepsy, although he also had a relaxed and patient disposition. He began lessons with Beethoven in 1804 and became not only an accomplished pianist but a composer as well. Although he remained devoted to Beethoven until the end, the composer seemed at times irritated by the archduke, and on a number of occasions excused himself on account of minor illness from lessons that had been previously arranged. To the archduke goes the honour not only of having the highest number of Beethoven's dedications but also some of the best of his compositions, including Piano Concertos nos. 4 and 5, two piano sonatas, the "Archduke" Piano Trio, op. 97, and above all the *Missa solemnis*, composed specifically for the archduke's enthronement as archbishop of Olmuz but not completed in time for the ceremonies.[117] It is curious that despite this apparent devotion, the archduke was absent from Beethoven's bedside during the composer's final illness.

In some ways Beethoven was spendthrift: for example, he frequently ate in taverns and would hire servants or horses on a whim.[118] He also was generous to those in need, and on a number of occasions he gave or sponsored benefit concerts for charitable institutions, orphans, and war widows.[119] His financial eccentricity is exemplified by his negotiating, and on a number of occasions even selling, compositions to more than one publisher. Because of his fame, his compositions were highly sought after and he used this knowledge in an attempt to maximize his revenue. In 1822, while completing the *Missa solemnis*, he was negotiating with at least four publishers simultaneously. To some he owed money, to others he promised one work and would deliver another, and on a number of occasions such conflicts led to litigation. These were difficult times for Beethoven, emotionally, physically, and financially. Thayer, always circumspect in his comments on Beethoven's occasional want of scruples, writes: "The conscientious reporter cannot ignore the actual, public facts and, hard as it is, cannot acquit Beethoven of the reproach that his conduct did not agree with the strict principles of honour and justice. These were dreary episodes in the history of Beethoven which nevertheless cannot be overlooked if he is to be wholly understood as a man."[120]

However, publishers also used provocative language in their letters to him. H.A. Probst, a publisher in Leipzig, offered to publish all Beethoven's works and was quite critical of his competitors, writing to Beethoven in 1824: "Unfortunately, pirate printing takes place everywhere. Already I see the highway robbers in Vienna waiting in ambush for your new works."[121] Publishers would alternately praise, cajole, and criticize him, and Beethoven, in turn, would play one off against another. Despite these feuds, and the publishers' offers of funds, the quality of his work was not affected adversely by his intrigues: he could easily, for example, have increased the quantity of his output to secure more money, but he did not do so. Beethoven frequently claimed poverty to justify the less-than-ethical management of his own finances, but he spent substantial sums on some things, including his frequent changes of residence and the legal expenses associated with his attempts to secure custody of his nephew. He was determined to bequeath an inheritance to his nephew, and was not poor at the time of his death.[122]

Beethoven lived in rented accommodation all his life and he rarely stayed long in one place, either because he became dissatisfied with the setting or because of a conflict with his landlord or his neighbours. Thayer lists a total of twenty-four different addresses in Vienna between 1792 and 1827.[123] His longest term of residence was four years (1810–14) at the Pasqualati House. In addition, from 1801 onward he spent every summer at a resort or spa in the countryside. His personal affairs and papers were known to be in a state of poorly concealed disorder, and he often worked on several compositions simultaneously. The marvel is that, despite the frequent moves of his belongings, he was able to maintain cohesion and continuity in compositions commonly completed years after they were begun. Beethoven also had endless disputes with his servants. His letters contain frequent disparaging references to their behaviour or attitudes. One example is a letter of complaint written in 1809 to his friend Nikolaus Zmeskall about a husband-and-wife employed as his servants; Beethoven ends by stating, "Both of them are wicked people."[124] (130) In two letters of 1818 to Frau Nanette Streicher (who by then had taken over the "management" of Beethoven's servants from Zmeskall), he vituperatively criticizes the servant's honesty, her "sweet tooth," and her morality. "What I have gone through with N[anni] far exceeds anything I have ever suffered from the many servants I have had,"[125] and "People of that type must be ruled not by affection but by fear. I threw half a dozen books at her. Probably one landed by chance on her brain or in her evil heart."[126]

TRANSITION PERIOD (1812–17)

The fracture of Beethoven's relationship with Antonie Brentano in 1812 marks the end of his second period music. The fact that he composed relatively little music during the following five years is perhaps a sign of inspirational exhaustion after the tremendously productive second period, but also, perhaps, a symptom of depression following the end of that relationship. In addition, the death of his brother Carl Caspar in 1815 was to have a powerful impact on Beethoven's health, emotional state, and creativity.

Carl had attempted a musical career and had done some teaching and composing. In 1802 (just before the Heiligenstadt Testament) he began acting as Beethoven's secretary and agent, negotiating with publishers and others, a role he continued until 1806 when he married Johanna. This situation may explain the affection that Beethoven displays toward Carl in the testament, while he was unable even to write the name of his other brother, Johann, in the same document. There were tensions between Beethoven and Carl, both of whom were hot-headed and stubborn, and on several occasions they even came to blows.[127] After his marriage, Carl obtained a lowly position as a government clerk and supplemented his salary by taking tenants in the house he owned with his wife. Carl and Johanna had only one son, Karl, born in 1806. In 1813 Carl developed tuberculosis, and although there was a brief remission by 1814, the disease recurred in 1815; he died in November of that year.

This event was seminal for Beethoven, not so much because of his brother's death but because of his ensuing battle with Carl's wife for custody of his nephew, Karl, a battle that lasted until early 1820 and consumed an enormous amount of Beethoven's energy and his physical and financial resources. During the years 1812–16, a barren period in his richly creative career, he also suffered a multitude of health problems that, while not life threatening, were unpleasant.

It was Carl's intention that Ludwig and Johanna have joint custody of the young Karl after Carl's death. He was aware of the tensions between his wife and his brother, and he reflected this awareness very touchingly in a codicil to his will:

I appoint my brother Ludwig van Beethoven guardian ... I ask, in full confidence and trust in his noble heart, that he shall bestow the love and friendship which he often showed me, upon my son Karl, and do all that is possible to promote the intellectual training and further welfare of my son. I know that he will not deny me this, my request. Having learned that my brother Hr. Ludwig van Beethoven, desires after my death to take wholly to himself my son Karl, and wholly to withdraw him from the supervision and training of his mother, and inasmuch as the best of harmony does not exist between my brother and my wife, I have found it necessary to add to my will that I by no means desire that my son be taken away from his mother, but that he shall always and so long as his future career permits remain with his mother, to which end the guardianship of him is to be exercised by her as well as my brother. Only by unity can the object which I had in view in appointing my brother guardian of my son, be attained, wherefore, for the welfare of my child, I recommend compliance to my wife and more moderation to my brother. God permit them to be harmonious for the sake of my child's welfare. This is the last wish of the dying husband and brother. Vienna, November 14, 1815 Carl van Beethoven.[128]

As will be seen from subsequent events, Beethoven paid little attention to his brother's wishes. Early in 1816, Beethoven won an initial lawsuit for custody and arranged for Karl, then age ten, to be sent to a private boarding school in Vienna. Beethoven then set about taking legal measures to prevent Johanna from visiting Karl at school. His correspondence reveals his extremely critical and judgmental attitude toward Johanna, whom he nicknamed "Queen of the Night" because of her reputation for loose moral standards.[129] He also took a stern line toward Karl, instructing Giannatasio, the school principal, to "hold him in strict obedience and if he does not obey you ... punish him at once."[130] Karl remained at the school until early 1818, when Beethoven took him home and engaged a private tutor. He was largely successful in ensuring that Karl rarely saw his mother, although they did manage to see each other on occasion when Johanna was able to bribe the servant while Beethoven was away. In mid-1818, she introduced proceedings to reclaim custody of her son, but her case was initially dismissed. The court allowed Beethoven to retain custody but, likely because of his unorthodox lifestyle and his deafness, insisted on the appointment of a co-guardian to act with Beethoven in the upbringing and education of the child. Beethoven was devastated in December

1818 when Karl ran away to be with his mother. Beethoven states that this event has driven him out of his mind,[131] but it did not lead him to consider Karl's emotional needs or his affection for his mother; on the contrary, Beethoven insisted even more strongly that the boy needed him and that if the boy was removed from his care there would be "disastrous consequences, both morally and politically."[132] Johanna appealed the decision, and in September 1819 the court granted guardianship of Karl to his mother, again with the appointment of a co-guardian. Beethoven in turn, with the support of his lawyer Johann Baptist Bach, prepared a detailed brief, and at an appeal court hearing in April 1820, won final custody of Karl.

Beethoven took up this custody battle against the advice of close friends such as Stephan von Breuning and Anton Schindler,[133] and he pursued it with determined tenacity, pulling every possible lever, including ethically questionable ones, to ensure that he won the case. For example, prior to the final court hearing in February 1820, he petitioned and communicated privately with the judge who was hearing the case.[134] While he won in the end, it was at great cost to his health, and also to his art, because of the music he did not compose during the three and a half years that he was preoccupied with the case. However, it is also conceivable that the emotional trauma accompanying his legal battles may have been instrumental in provoking the change in style that led to the music of his late period.

His many health problems during this period are often couched in general terms: "I have been in very poor health, so much so that I have thought of my death" [May 1816];[135] and "I have been in bed for eight days" [November 1816].[136] At times he also specifies a chest complaint [July 1816],[137] a "feverish cold" [February 1817],[138] anxiety and depression [June 1817],[139] and distress about his hearing loss [July 1817].[140] In July 1817 his physician Dr Staudenheim diagnosed "a disease of the lungs,"[141] and shortly thereafter Beethoven wrote to his friend Nikolaus Zmeskall: "I often despair and I would like to die."[142] His respiratory symptoms, including cough, colds, and "chills," continued into 1818, after which time they diminished.

Beethoven had a distinctive attitude to his health and a strongly ambivalent relationship with his physicians. He was not only concerned about his health problems, such as deafness and gastro-intestinal symptoms, but also took an active part in seeking treatment and attempting to heal. He read widely about health issues and was aware of and willing to experiment with new treatments such as galvanism and Brunonianism. We know of at least eleven physicians who treated him during his lifetime (their backgrounds and areas of interest are discussed in chapter 3). He sought them out because of their reputations and expertise and initially would be compliant with their recommendations, but would become critical, disgruntled, and even patronizing if his condition was not "cured." He would follow their drug recommendations up to a point, but often took more than the suggested dose in the belief that this improved effectiveness. Throughout his life he retained a strong belief in the effectiveness of water spa treatment. Early in 1826, during the final full year of his life, he lost the support of Dr Braunhofer, and for a ten-month period, even though he was ailing, he did not have a physician. With the onset of his final illness in December Holz and Schindler had to scramble to find a new physician, because his previous doctors all declined, for various reasons, to attend him. It was thus that Dr Wawruch came to care for him during the final three and a half months of his life.

The care of Karl and the accompanying custody battle caused Beethoven great anxiety. In a letter to his friend Nanette Streicher he complains bitterly and at length about his servants who seemingly were colluding with Karl behind his back to enable the boy to visit with his mother, accusing them of "treachery."[143] He ends by saying, "This affair has given me a dreadful heart attack from which I have not yet completely recovered." Although he was pleased and relieved by his eventual victory, it was not the end of his anxieties about Karl. Difficulties and conflicts continued until the onset of the composer's final illness in December 1826. Beethoven's relationship with Karl was complex. Although legally the boy was his nephew, he regarded him as his son and often addressed him or spoke of him as such, particularly in his later years.[144] While he undoubtedly felt genuine, fatherly affection toward Karl, his relentless pursuit of legal guardianship, and his stern criticism of the moral ineptitude of Johanna, suggest that he saw himself as being on a rescue mission to protect his young nephew from falling under what he regarded as her evil spell. At times he adopted a paternalistic and judgmental attitude toward Karl.

Editha Sterba and Richard Sterba have examined the triangular relationship between Beethoven, Carl (his brother), and Karl (his nephew) from the psychoanalytic perspective. After reviewing the composer's relationship with Carl, they conclude that it was "too intimate, too blind, too indulgent and too emotional – the unconscious homosexual factor is unmistakable."[145] They also refer to a "strong unconscious homosexual component" in Beethoven's relationship with several of his friends, including Amenda, Tremont, and Holz,[146] but they do not suggest an active homosexual relationship between the composer and any of these individuals. The authors note that after the final settlement of the custody issue, Karl became attached to Beethoven and took on the latter's attitudes and prejudices. However, he remained a lively, engaging, and intelligent youth, and was even able, at times, to speak his mind affirmatively toward his strong-minded uncle.

In 1825, Karl attended the Polytechnic School in Vienna and while there received many letters from Beethoven. These include not only expressions of love and tenderness but also negative tirades, criticism, and exhortations. This intensely ambivalent quality to their relationship continued through 1826, with conflicts over money, studies, and Karl's future. Karl felt increasingly trapped, and this situation no doubt triggered the serious crisis in their relationship that occurred in 1826.

THE THIRD VIENNA (MATURE) PERIOD.

The custody decision of 1820 finally freed Beethoven from a perceived Sword of Damocles and allowed him to actively resume composing. His third period was inaugurated in 1818 with the publication of the Piano Sonata in B flat major, op. 106 ("Hammerklavier"), a work he had begun the previous year. During his remaining years, despite his increasingly severe deafness, he was to compose some of the most profound, sublime music ever written, including the *Missa solemnis*, op. 123, the Symphony no. 9, op. 125, the last four piano sonatas (op. 106, 109, 110, and 111), the

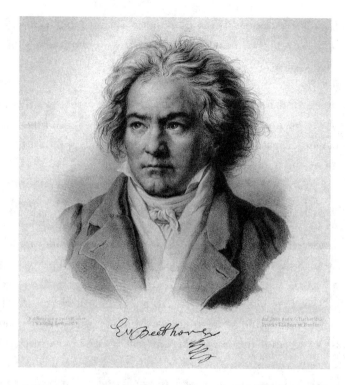

Lithograph of Beethoven by C. Fischer, based on an undated drawing by August von Klöber (1793–1864), likely made during Beethoven's third Vienna period. Ira F. Brilliant Center for Beethoven Studies, San José State University, CA.

Diabelli Variations, op. 120, and the last five string quartets (op. 130, 131, 132, 133, and 135).

Some authors, including Thayer,[147] comment on Beethoven's loose and variable connection with the Catholic church, in which he was baptized and brought up. Although it is not known whether he attended church services and sacraments regularly, he did write prayers in the *Tagebuch*. In these prayers he is preoccupied with his suffering, his isolation and guilt, and his relationship with Karl: "God help me, Thou seest me deserted by all men, for I do not wish to do wrong, hear my supplication, but to be with my Karl in the future when now no possibility can be found. Oh harsh fate, Oh cruel destiny, no, no, my unhappy condition will never end ... God, God, my refuge my rock, my all, Thou seest my inmost heart and knowest how it pains me to be obliged to compel another to suffer by my good labors for my precious Karl!!!! O hear me always, Thou Ineffable One hear me – thy unhappy, most unhappy of mortals."[148] In the Conversation Books he states, "Socrates and Jesus are my models."[149] His letters also contain frequent references to God and divine intervention.[150] Von Breuning refers to Beethoven's "ideal" faith in God,[151] and Schmidt-Gorg describes him as being attached to the church for his lifetime.[152]

The music Beethoven wrote during this final period can best be summed up as introspective, and these works also have a powerful spiritual undertone that is evident not only in the texts of the *Missa solemnis* and the "Ode to Joy," but also in the depth and range of the musical forms in the final sonatas and string quartets. Although there are moments of tension and agitation in these works, one senses a search for peace, serenity, and meaning in his life.

It is appropriate to question why and how Beethoven could compose music of this nature when his body was wracked with illness, his mind preoccupied with the continued cares and turmoil of daily life, and not a single note he wrote was audible to him. The answer must be that he was searching for, and had finally found, an inner peace, and that through his music he was communicating with his Maker. His very deafness and the accompanying social isolation forced him to look inward and to depend only on himself. This was his way of communicating with his God and with the world, and fortunately for us all, his natural genius – accompanied by the extent and breadth of his musical training – enabled him to internalize sound, so that he could still "hear" what he was writing. These final works transcend emotion and words.

The last seven years were marked also by serious health problems and continuing difficulties in his relationship with Karl. In August of 1821, he developed an attack of painless jaundice that lasted six weeks, which he mentions briefly in two letters to Archduke Rudolf: "I had been very

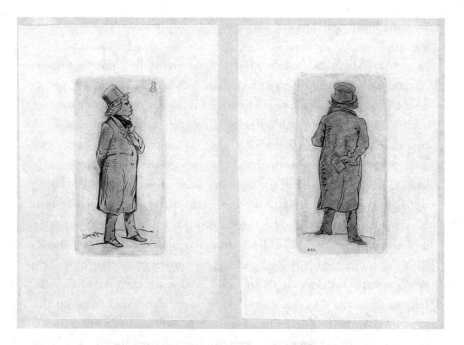

These two depictions by Joseph Böhm show Beethoven, ca 1820, in characteristic posture, walking in the street carrying his notebook. Beethoven-Haus, Bonn.

poorly for a long time when finally jaundice definitely set in; and in my case it seems to be an extremely objectionable disease."[153] As part of his convalescence, he went to Baden. One day he went for a long walk in the countryside dressed in very casual clothes. He became lost after darkness set in and seems to have behaved inappropriately, drawing the attention of the police, who arrested him as a tramp. Upon being informed by the "tramp" that he was Beethoven, the policeman responded, "Of course, why not? You're a tramp: Beethoven doesn't look so," and marched him off to the cell for the night. When Beethoven continued to agitate, in the middle of the night the police commissioner called a musical director who lived in the neighborhood to come and identify him. The director, as soon as he set eyes on him, confirmed that this was Beethoven. The Police

Commissioner apologized, and Beethoven went home with the musical director.[154]

In 1822 Anton Schindler (1795–1864) became Beethoven's unpaid secretary and from then on assumed an increasingly important role in Beethoven's life. Schindler also became Beethoven's principal caregiver during his final illness. Schindler had trained as a lawyer but was also a competent violinist and conductor. He became acquainted with Beethoven after 1816, and, since he worked in the office of Johann Bach, Beethoven's lawyer, he was involved in the custody battle for Karl. After becoming Beethoven's secretary, his attitude toward the composer became obsequious. He quoted, with approval, the following statement made by someone he considered an "enemy" of Beethoven, who described his relationship with the composer thus: "Schindler gave himself to Beethoven as one gives oneself to the Devil: body and soul. He stayed; others were less faithful, and gradually the great artist found himself alone. He was eventually abandoned by his best and oldest friends, and only a few of them gathered at his deathbed."[155] Beethoven both used and abused him in return. In letters to Schindler he addressed him as "Papagano" and "Samothracian scoundrel."[156] In March 1825, Schindler was supplanted as Beethoven's friend, secretary, and amanuensis by Karl Holz, another amateur violinist. Schindler was offended by this situation and his jealousy led him to subsequent criticisms of Holz. After Beethoven's death Schindler criticized Holz for spreading rumors – false, in his opinion – that Beethoven was a drunkard. Schindler returned to Beethoven's favour only in December 1826 with the onset of the composer's final illness and he cared for him faithfully until the end. He also collected Beethoven's papers after his death and published a biography of the composer in 1840.[157] Although this monograph is an invaluable resource, it also reflects Schindler's sycophantic attitude, and he has been criticized severely for destroying invaluable documents, including portions of the Conversation Books, probably because their content did not support his view of Beethoven.[158]

In 1822, Beethoven was again preoccupied with financial problems. His medical, legal, and residential expenses were high and his revenues reduced, partly because of his deep involvement with large, time-

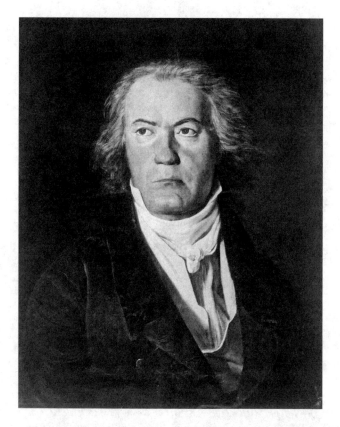

*In this portrait by Ferdinand Waldmüller, made in 1823,
Beethoven, aged about fifty-two, appears introspective and
prematurely aged. By this time he had suffered his first attack of
liver failure, and his deafness was far advanced.
Beethoven-Haus, Bonn.*

consuming works such as the *Missa solemnis* and the Symphony no. 9,
and partly because of a reduction in the pensions he received from some
of his more affluent admirers. He also owed money to several publishers.
In order to restore financial order he attempted to borrow money from his
brother Johann,[159] who by this time was well off: his apothecary business

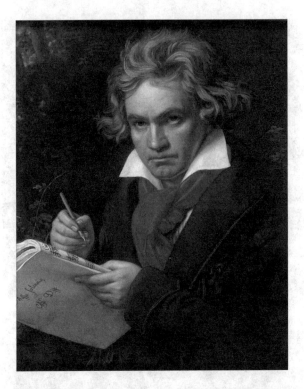

Painting of Beethoven composing the Missa Solemnis, *1820,
by Joseph Stieler (1781–1858); the word "Credo" can be seen
on the manuscript. Beethoven-Haus, Bonn.*

had prospered, and he enjoyed his property. The appeal for a loan brought
Johann back into Beethoven's life. Despite his reputation for parsimony,
he agreed to a loan, but the amount is not known. Beethoven was also able
to publish some smaller pieces (the eleven bagatelles, op. 119) and in 1823,
as the *Missa solemnis* neared completion, he delayed its publication in
order to invite most of the royal houses in Europe along with a number of
other illustrious individuals to subscribe to the project. In return for their
subscription, they were to receive an autographed copy of the publication.

The *Missa solemnis* was originally intended for performance in 1820 at the installation of Archduke Rudolf as archbishop of Olmuz, but at the time of the installation the work was nowhere near completion. It was finally completed in 1823 but the premiere was delayed until March 1824 when it was performed in Vienna along with the Sympony no. 9. Although it is a dramatic rather than a religious work, the *Missa solemnis* nevertheless reflects Beethoven's deep spirituality;[160] it has been described as the "Voice of God"[161] and has also been used to symbolize peace by the organization International Physicians for the Prevention of Nuclear War, a group that received the Nobel Peace Prize in 1985.[162]

The Symphony no. 9, op. 125, is Beethoven's best-known work from this period and is perhaps one of the greatest orchestral compositions of all time. It was likely conceived in 1821 when Beethoven was well into work on the *Missa solemnis*. The setting of Schiller's "Ode to Joy" in the final movement is the first occasion in music history that voices are used in a symphonic form. By 1824, when the new symphony was ready for performance, Beethoven had become disenchanted with Vienna and the musical appreciation of its citizens, and had begun negotiations to have the premiere in Berlin. On hearing of this, a group of thirty leading Viennese citizens, led by Prince Lichnowsky, wrote to Beethoven pleading to have the first performance in Vienna. Beethoven responded appreciatively and affirmatively and the concert took place in March 1824. It was during this performance that a famous incident took place. At the completion of the symphony, the audience broke out in thunderous applause; Beethoven, who was at the front of the auditorium facing the orchestra, had to be physically turned around to see the applause he could not hear.[163]

In 1823, Beethoven developed problems with his eyes – predominantly bilateral pain accompanied at times by photophobia, but seemingly without discharge or lacrimation. These symptoms are first mentioned cursorily in April;[164] a month later in a postscript to Anton Schindler, he writes: "My eyes, which are rather worse than better, allow me to see everything only very slowly,"[165] and, "For a whole three weeks I had in addition sore eyes and by doctor's orders I was forbidden to write or read."[166] In two letters he complains that town air aggravates his eye symptoms,[167] and he mentions them on one final occasion in January 1824.[168] Beethoven's general health remained poor. He went to the spa at Baden in September, from where he writes: "I arrived here in a very sick condition. For my health is very shaky,"[169] and "My doctor assured me yesterday that I really am recovering from my illness. But I must still take a whole bottle of mixture in 24 hours and, as it is a purgative, I find the treatment very weakening ... you will see from the enclosed instructions given by my doctor that I have to take a good deal of exercise." In June 1825, he also had a premonition of death, writing to Karl, "Death with his scythe will not spare me very much longer."[170]

Some of his visitors provided him with lighthearted relief. Caroline Unger, a twenty-year-old singer who visited on several occasions teases Beethoven about coming to live with him as his cook, and says, "You must marry – an old boy is a useless citizen ... Dixi et sanavi animam meam." (I have spoken and have saved my soul).[171] A few days later she visited him again.[172] Beethoven must have asked her if she had a lover, and she replies, "No, I do not have one – how many lovers have you had?" Unfortunately we do not have Beethoven's reply. During a visit three months later, Caroline teases him again, calling him "lazy" because he did not accept an invitation to go to a recital with her, and chaffs him for making eyes at another young woman – "The pretty eyes of my friend could become dangerous" – at which Beethoven laughs.[173]

By 1824 Karl had become the equivalent of his secretary, and over the next twelve to eighteen months Beethoven dictated many of his letters to him. By then their relationship had become curiously intense and ambivalent. Beethoven attempted to control Karl's activities and friendships. For example, Karl had developed a close friendship with a young man called Niemetz. Beethoven disapproved of Niemetz and attempted strenuously to persuade Karl to break off this relationship but Karl stood his ground, writing that he had known Niemetz for four years and that he was like a brother to him.[174] Karl comes through as "lively, clever, and shrewd," and he was able to exploit his knowledge of Beethoven to his own advantage.[175] Karl could also be affectionate and would call him *bester* ("dear fellow" or "old boy").[176] In 1825, however, there were increasing conflicts

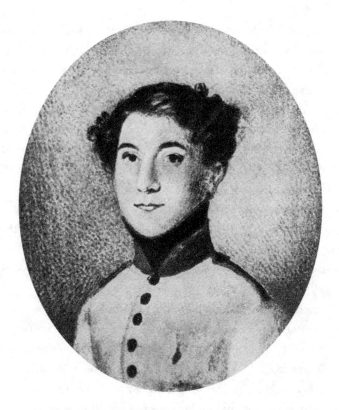

*Beethoven's nephew Karl van Beethoven at age nineteen,
about the time of the composer's death. Beethoven won custody
of Karl in 1820 after a three-year custody battle, but he had a rather
complex and ambivalent relationship with the boy. The image
reproduces a miniature produced in the nineteenth-century
by an unknown artist. Beethoven-Haus, Bonn.*

over Karl's future career and his continued visits to his mother. Beethoven
tried every ruse to prevent these visits, including angry outbursts in which
he accused his nephew of lies and selfishness: "It is my wish that your self-
ish behaviour to be shall cease once and for all."[177] However, most of his
letters are full of love and affection: "I embrace and kiss you a thousand

times, not as my prodigal son, but as my newly born son," and "Write me a few words – send them to me tomorrow. Here is another florin, don't forget to bathe – keep well. Take care of yourself so that you do not fall ill ... Be my dear son."[178]

Beethoven's fame attracted a steady stream of visitors from all parts of Europe who wished to pay their respects, but as far as we know, there was only one visitor from the New World. In 1825 Théodore Frédéric Molt, a music teacher in Quebec, made a pilgrimage to Vienna and wrote the following note in Beethoven's Conversation Book: "I am a music teacher in Quebec, in North America. Your works have delighted me so often that I consider it my duty to pay you my personal gratitude on a journey through Vienna." A few days later Molt wrote to Beethoven, asking him to write a brief canon as a memento "from his great soul," which Beethoven obligingly did.[179]

By 1826, Beethoven's behaviour was becoming increasingly inappropriate, and both the conflicts with Karl and his health problems grew more serious. He spoke in a loud voice, used animated gestures, and had a loud, ringing laugh.[180] He would expectorate in the room and seriously neglected his appearance and behaviour. By mid-1826 the conflicts with Karl reached a crisis point. Beethoven was angered by what he perceived as his nephew's laziness, his tendency to gamble and spend money inappropriately, and his indecision about his future. Karl, on the other hand, resented his uncle's attempts to control his life: "You ask me why I do not talk ... (it is) because I have had enough ... yours is the right to command, and I must endure it all."[181] Late in July, he pawned his watch for two pistols, went to some old ruins near Baden, and discharged both toward his head. One missed completely, and the other caused superficial scalp abrasions. A passing workman discovered him some hours later; Karl asked to be taken to his mother's house, where Beethoven eventually found him. In response to Beethoven's questions, he wrote, "Do not plague me with reproaches and lamentations; it is past. Later all matters may be adjusted."[182] At that time attempted suicide was a crime; in answer to police questioning as to why he had done it, Karl replied that his uncle "tormented me too much," and "I grew worse because my uncle wanted me to be better."[183] In a note to Beethoven in 1823 foreshadowing his suicide attempt, Karl refers to an actor, Kustner, who got into financial difficulties and shot himself, adding: "Here (in Vienna) suicide is not as common as in Paris. There, when you have lost everything, you go to the firearms merchant where you can rent a pistol with your remaining coins."[184] This is almost exactly what Karl did three years later in similar circumstances.

In psychiatric terms, it seems likely that Karl's suicide attempt was a gesture, a "cry for help," when he found himself in an increasingly caged situation. He may also have been depressed, but there is no evidence that he had serious psychiatric pathology either before or after this event. Although his attempt was elaborately planned – buying pistols, writing farewell letters, travelling to a secluded country spot – it is difficult to believe that Karl was such a poor shot that he could not have taken better aim at his brain, unless there was a large part of him that did not wish to die. The motives of individuals who attempt but do not complete suicide are commonly mixed, and a large segment is a vicarious attempt to resolve a problem. In Karl's case, his problem was a need to establish more self-sufficiency and individuality and to escape from the overpowering shadow of his uncle. In effect, his suicide attempt did solve these problems, although not immediately. After a six-week hospitalization, Karl returned home with Beethoven who, after some initial resistance, agreed with Karl's decision to join the Austrian army as a cadet. His application was accepted; all that remained was to allow time for the disfiguring wound to heal and his hair to grow back. In the fall of 1826 Beethoven accepted a long-standing invitation from his brother Johann to spend a few months, accompanied by Karl, at Johann's estate at Gneixendorf, about sixty kilometers from Vienna. Local peasants would see Beethoven walking in the fields, gesticulating, singing, and ignoring people, even the servants and peasants who were laughing at him. At the same time, he was completing his final work, the sublime String Quartet in F major, op. 135.[185] On the whole, the two-month stay at Gneixendorf was tranquil and productive.

He went for long walks in the fields, always with his notebook to write down his musical ideas, and he completed movements of two string quartets while there. These were his final compositions.

However there were also moments of conflict both between the brothers and between Beethoven and Karl. Since Beethoven showed little enthusiasm for returning to Vienna, Johann eventually wrote him a letter, stating that Karl was becoming increasingly indolent and pointing out Beethoven's duty to return to Vienna to allow Karl to pursue his career in the army.

BEETHOVEN'S FINAL ILLNESS

Beethoven and Karl left Gneixendorf for Vienna on 1 December 1826, spending a night *en voyage* in a cold and draughty house, and arriving back at Beethoven's home the following day. Dr Wawruch, Beethoven's physician during his final illness, gives the following description of this journey:

That December was raw, damp, cold and frosty; Beethoven's clothing anything but adapted to the unfriendly season of the year, and yet he was urged on by an eternal unrest and a gloomy foreboding of misfortune. He was compelled to spend a night in a village tavern where, besides wretched shelter, he found an unwarmed room without winter shutters. Toward midnight he experienced his first fever-chill, a dry hacking cough accompanied by violent thirst and cutting pains in the side. When seized with the fever he drank a few measures of ice-cold water and longed, helplessly, for the first rays of the morning light. Weak and ill, he permitted himself to be lifted into the *Leiterwagen* and arrived, at last, weak, exhausted and without strength in Vienna.[186]

Dr Braunhofer, Beethoven's regular doctor, declined to attend him, ostensibly because it was too far for him to go. However Walter Nohl, the author of a book discussing the relationship between Braunhofer and Beethoven, speculates that Braunhofer knew that this was likely Beethoven's terminal illness and had no desire to be in charge at the time of his death.[187] Beethoven's friend Karl Holz managed to recruit Dr Wawruch, who came to see him on 5 December, three days after the return from Gneixendorf. At his first visit Wawruch introduced himself by saying, "I am a great admirer of yours and will do everything possible to help."[188] Marek reports that the remaining pages of the Conversation Book containing Wawruch's introductory interview with Beethoven have been torn out, presumably by Schindler.[189] After his examination, Wawruch concluded:

I found Beethoven afflicted with serious symptoms of inflammation of the lungs, his face glowed, he spat blood, his respiration threatened suffocation and a painful stitch in the side made lying on the back a torment. A severe counter-treatment for inflammation soon brought the desired relief; his constitution triumphed and by a lucky crisis he was freed from apparent mortal danger, so that on the fifth day he was able, in a sitting posture, to tell me, amid profound emotion, of the discomforts he has suffered. On the seventh day he felt considerably better, so that he was able to get out of bed, walk about, read and write.

During these seven days from 5 to 12 December, Beethoven composed four letters (written by Karl at Beethoven's dictation): a letter to Karl Holz stating that he was so ill that he had to stay in bed and asking Holz to visit him,[190] a long and affectionate letter to Franz Wegeler in Bonn, in reply to Wegeler's letter written the previous year,[191] and two business letters to publishers. In each of these letters, he makes reference to being ill and in bed but provides no further details.

Based on both Wawruch's and Beethoven's reports, it is probable that Beethoven had a form of pneumonia, the symptoms of which are cough, fever, hemoptysis (blood in the sputum), dyspnea (breathlessness), and pleurisy (inflammation of the membranes surrounding the lungs causing the pain in his side). Prior to antibiotics, pneumonia commonly lasted a week to ten days; recovery, when it occurred, was preceded by a "crisis." Breuning believed that Beethoven had an attack of peritonitis, but this is improbable: the symptoms do not fit, and moreover, he would not likely have survived this condition in the pre-antibiotic era.[192] However a few days later a new and more serious problem developed: a recurrence of jaundice, indicating that liver failure had begun. Wawruch noted that the liver had "hard knots," and his diagnosis was "dropsy," a generic term used to describe the accumulation of fluid in the legs, abdomen, and lower back. While dropsy can occur in heart, kidney, or liver disease, the method by which the fluid accumulates differs according to the underlying cause. In liver failure, the fluid accumulation is caused either by mechanical constriction of the main vein that returns blood from the legs and abdomen to the heart as it passes through the liver, or by biochemical changes in the blood resulting from liver failure: the blood can no longer hold the fluid within the blood vessels and seeps out into the tissues.

Other symptoms and signs mentioned by Wawruch are vomiting, diarrhea (*Brechdurchfall*), violent rage, trembling, and shivering. Beethoven also was "bent double" because of the pains; there was lessened "segregation" of the urine; and he experienced "nocturnal suffocation." Liver failure, in and of itself, is not usually accompanied by pain. Since gallstones were found at autopsy, it is conceivable that he was suffering attacks of biliary colic resulting from blockage of the bile duct by stones; this would have further aggravated the jaundice. Another possible cause of the pain is pancreatitis. The attack of violent rage accompanied by trembling and shivering and the "threatening mental tempest" may have been caused by emotional frustration accompanying his illness, or it may have been a manifestation of hepatic encephalopathy. The "nocturnal suffocation" was likely the result of the abdominal fluid pressing on the diaphragm, causing physical restriction of respiratory expansion.

Dr Wawruch had consulted with Dr Staudenheim (one of Beethoven's former physicians), who agreed that paracentesis (removal of fluid from the abdominal cavity by insertion of a needle or a tube) was indicated, and Beethoven underwent this procedure on 20 December. The operation was performed by Dr Seibert. As the tube was inserted and the water spurted out, Beethoven said: "Professor, you remind me of Moses striking the rock with his staff."[193] Dr Wawruch stated that "the liquid amounted to twenty-five pounds but the after flow was certainly five times as much." This represents a huge quantity – one wonders if his measurements were correct. Substantial symptomatic relief followed the release of the fluid.[194] Beethoven's condition improved somewhat over the next few days but the fluid gradually re-accumulated in his abdomen. A second operation was performed on 8 January. Beethoven had two further tappings of fluid in his abdomen on 2 and 27 February, again performed by Dr Seibert. While the first had been accompanied by an infection at the site of the wound, the remaining three appear to have been uncomplicated. Although each brought some symptomatic relief, the improvement was less each time, and the fluid in the abdomen returned because the underlying mechanism of its production was unresolved.

Karl Holz, who had been Beethoven's friend, associate, and secretary for the previous eighteen months, married about this time; for this and perhaps other reasons, he largely passed out of Beethoven's life, allowing Schindler to regain his previous close relationship with the composer. Beethoven, however, must have voiced his apprehensions about being discarded again by Schindler, for we find Schindler saying on 18 December: "I protest for the thousandth time that I will never abandon you." Schindler expressed his dismay about Holz's "many intrigues," and added "That's why I came so rarely. Nevertheless, I responded immediately to your written requests. What is the point of my advice if the chatter of Holz, Karl and your brother neutralize everything. [Stephan von] Breuning and Bernard are also fed up. The behaviour of certain people around you is like oriental princes – (you are) Sultan Beethoven."

These brief but telling extracts reflect the intrigues and personality clashes swirling around Beethoven's entourage at the onset of his terminal illness. Clearly, Schindler had been upset that Holz, Karl, and Johann had usurped his previous close association with Beethoven. He assures Beethoven that he, Breuning, and other friends will resume their support for him, but only if Holz, Karl, and Johann pass out of the picture. This, in fact, is what happened. Holz married and Johann, who lived outside Vienna, had little to do with his brother until the final weeks. Karl left Vienna on 2 January 1827 to join the army as a cadet, and never saw Beethoven again. The following day, Beethoven dictated his will to his lawyer, nominating Karl as his sole heir and Stephan von Breuning as

Karl's surrogate father. His remaining letters were all written by Anton Schindler to Beethoven's dictation.

Early in February, Johann Stumpff, a friend who was living in London, sent Beethoven a forty-volume set of George Frideric Handel's works. This gave Beethoven great pleasure, as he had a very high regard for Handel. In his letter of gratitude he describes his poor health and financial difficulties, and asks his London friends to arrange a benefit concert on his behalf.[195] It is clear from the brief and affectionate letters to Wegeler and Zmeskall dictated on 17 and 18 February that his condition was deteriorating.[196] He remained bedridden and weak, although there were fleeting moments of optimism. For example, on 6 March he states: "If this continues, my illness will last until the middle of summer,"[197] and on 17 March (only ten days before his death, after a consultation with his former physician, Dr Malfatti): "Truly a miracle … thanks to Malfatti's skill my life is being saved."[198]

Details of his medical treatments during the final three months are derived mainly from Wawruch's report and from those sections of the Conversation Books that have been preserved. The latter contain revealing questions and comments put to Beethoven by Schindler, Stephan von Breuning and his son Gerhard, the physicians who attended him, and visitors who came during his final illness.[199]

Schindler [1 January 1827]: "Wawruch knows his business and is a respected physician."

[5 January] "Do you still have a good appetite?" "Dr Seibert wants to delay the second operation – this is preferable to preventing a third." "Do not lose confidence in your doctor – he already has done a lot because dropsy takes a long time to cure." "Must I be here with your doctor?" "No" [replies Beethoven].

[25 January] "The mother of a friend has recommended a recipe for you … an infusion of juniper berries followed by cabbage, caraway seeds and hay flower. The doctors will say no, naturally."

[2 February, after a third operation]: "I wonder if you would like [Dr] Malfatti to come today to see the state of your liver and stomach … The good function of the liver is necessary to restore your health. Malfatti can perhaps give some better advice ... also he likes and admires you ... he complimented me on my report about you which was as good as one of his assistants ... He agrees with Wawruch's approach ... he wants you to get out of bed as soon as possible and take this prescription and also the wine ... when this dose of Gumbold's kirschner is finished there is more for you in his cellar."

[Late February or early March]: "[Holz] recently told Breuning that by midday you have drunk more than a measure of wine, and other lies."

At this point there is an annotation in the margin that Prod'homme identifies as having been written by Schindler at a later date: "One must observe here that after the death of Beethoven, Holz was the only one who went about saying openly, everywhere, that Beethoven had contracted dropsy because he drank too much wine; thence the view spread that he had become a drunkard. The truth is that Holz himself was a big drinker, and on several occasions enticed Beethoven to drink more than usual. But God be praised, the period during which he let himself be led by Holz and drank a lot lasted only about eighteen months, from the beginning of summer 1825 to the end of September 1826."

Stephan von Breuning [February 1827]: "Schindler is very attached to you. I like him more than that egoist Holz ... you must not become emotional, you must only think of pleasant things as this helps recovery."

Gerhard von Breuning [20 February 1827]: "It is now three days since you had anything to eat ... it must be *vin nouveau* – it is so tart that it contracts the mouth – it has already gone off ... no one can stand Holz, all who know him say he is false ... He pretends that he likes you a lot – he is a hypocrite and he lies like a book. You are the best of men and all the others are rascals. It's only your wine that he likes." "You seem to be very tired today. You and father [Stephan] should go together to a water spa this summer. On the whole your spirits don't seem to be weak. Is your stomach still sore? When there is no bandage, the wound gets inflamed. I heard it said today that bedbugs bothered you when you were sleeping. Sleep is good for you. I'll bring something to chase away the bedbugs. Tell the doctor that you must eat meat."

[27 February 1827]: "I hope that I am not tiring you with my chatter. Wolfmayer likes you a lot. When he left he said with tears in his eyes, 'The great man, alas, alas!' He asked if you still had some wine."

[28 February 1827]: "Dr Malfatti is your best doctor; also he likes you a lot. He will certainly come to see you again. He does not bother at all if you take a few bottles of wine. It does not make him any richer and he desires only to make you better. I will come back tonight at 7.15 if it does not bother you."

Judging from these exchanges, it is clear that Gerhard had a friendly, engaging relationship with Beethoven. He not only asked questions about his health but also chattered about literature, travel, and other topics. Beethoven enjoyed his visits, and gave Gerhard the affectionate nickname of "Hosenknopf" (pants button).[200] It is a touching coincidence that in his youth Beethoven was "mothered" by Stephan von Breuning's mother, and on his deathbed he was supported and succored by Breuning's thirteen-year-old son. In due course, Gerhard von Breuning himself became a physician, and in later life wrote a biography of Beethoven[201] in which he is critical of the physicians who treated Beethoven in his final illness. He states that Dr Wawruch's treatments had done nothing for the "underlying cause," and that this had led to the accumulation of abdominal fluid.[202] He also disapproved of the tapping carried out by Dr Seibert because the skin around the wound became inflamed.[203] He states that even Beethoven became disenchanted with Wawruch's "dry mercenary attitude," and on several occasions broke into a "violent tirade" against him. Gerhard is also critical of Dr Malfatti, whom Wawruch consulted and reports that Beethoven called Malfatti an "ass."[204]

There is no reason to doubt Gerhard's descriptions of Beethoven's critical attitude to his physicians. Beethoven had a long history of this, and had exhausted the patience and reserves of a number of their predecessors. However, Gerhard von Breuning's condemnation of Wawruch and Malfatti is unjustified. They offered the best that was available in early nineteenth-century medicine. Beethoven was in terminal liver failure, and even in the early twenty-first century, physicians would have had difficulty managing his case. Going to the "root cause" of his problem, as von

Breuning rightly recommends, would have meant removing the causes of the liver failure and restoring the hepatic function – assuming that they were able to correctly diagnose the condition. In present-day medicine, an individual with Beethoven's type of liver failure would likely require a liver transplant.

After Karl's departure for the army, Anton Schindler became Beethoven's main support and caregiver, and he made valiant efforts to maintain Beethoven's confidence in his physicians. About Dr Wawruch he states: "I have a great deal of confidence in him ... he is known as an able man – esteemed and appreciated by his students ... my advice from the beginning has been to take into consultation a physician whose familiarity with your constitution comes from medical treatment,"[205] and "Yesterday I urged your brother earnestly to hold a medical council of men who have known your constitution longer ... Staudenheim, Braunhofer, and Malfatti, three men whose judgment is not to be rejected."[206] Subsequently, Schindler became critical of Wawruch, and successfully effected a reconciliation between Beethoven and Dr Malfatti (who had been Beethoven's physician ten years previously). Schindler managed to persuade Wawruch to bring in Malfatti as a consultant, although Malfatti made it clear that he was leaving Wawruch in charge of the case. Following a "council of physicians" on 11 January, it was recommended that Beethoven be given frozen fruit punch and that his abdomen be rubbed with ice-cold water.[207] Wawruch described the results of this approach:

Dr Malfatti, who thenceforth supported me with his advice, and who, as a friend of Beethoven's of long years' standing, understood his predominant inclination for spirituous liquors, hit upon the notion of administering frozen punch. I must confess that the treatment produced excellent results for a few days at least. Beethoven felt himself so refreshed by the ice with its alcoholic contents that already in the first night he slept quietly throughout the night and began to perspire profusely. He grew cheerful and was full of witty comments ... But this joy ... did not last. He began to abuse the prescription and applied himself right bravely to the frozen punch. The spirits soon caused a violent pressure of the blood upon the brain; he grew soporous, breathed stertorously like an intoxicated person, began to wander in his speech, and a few times inflammatory pains in the throat were paired with hoarseness and even aphony. He became more unruly, and when, because of a cooling of the bowels, colic and diarrhea resulted, it was high time to deprive him of this precious refreshment.

Despite his disapproval of Wawruch, Schindler admitted that the frozen punch had had a beneficial effect, but he accused Wawruch of "making defamatory remarks [about Beethoven] which glossed over his poor [medical] treatment."[208] Despite his many faults, Schindler was Beethoven's most loyal and devoted caregiver during his final illness. He spared no effort to ensure his "master's" comfort, and attempted to smooth Beethoven's relationship with his physicians, his family, and the world. Schindler's devotion was so complete that at one point it appears that he developed what now would be called "caregiver burnout." On 27 February he wrote to Moscheles (a friend of Beethoven's who at that time lived in London):

What hurts him greatly is the fact that no one here takes any notice of him; and in truth this lack of interest is striking. Formerly people drove up in their carriages if he were no more than indisposed; now he is totally forgotten, as though he had never lived in Vienna. I myself suffer the greater annoyance, and earnestly wish that matters may soon take a turn with him, in one or other way, for I am losing all my time since I devote it altogether to him, because he will suffer none other about him, and to abandon him in his absolutely helpless condition would be inhuman.[209]

The combination of avoidance of the sick person by some and exhaustion of those who attend and provide care is not uncommon in situations of severe or terminal illness.

In late January 1827, Beethoven was given hot baths with a view to stimulating perspiration, but this had no beneficial effect. Schindler reported that Wawruch was "ruining him with too much medicine,"[210] and that he had "emptied seventy-five bottles, without counting various powders." Little is known about the content of these medicines, but most were likely what would now be called herbal or naturopathic remedies. We do know that he was given almond milk, a salep drink, and juniper berry tea.

By early February it was becoming clear that Beethoven had serious liver problems. On 2 February Schindler reported (presumably having obtained information from the physicians) that Dr Malfatti would check his liver and belly, and that "the well-being of the liver is the key to the whole sickness."[211] However, after the fourth tapping on 27 February, Beethoven became very depressed. Wawruch reported "no words of comfort could brace him up, and when I promised him alleviation of his sufferings with the coming of the vitalizing weather of spring, he answered with a smile, 'My day's work is finished. If there were a physician who could help me his name shall be called 'Wonderful.' This pathetic allusion to Handel's *Messiah* touched me so deeply that I had to confess its correctness to myself with profound emotion." During February Beethoven also had affectionate correspondence with two old friends, Franz Wegeler (still in Bonn) and Nikolaus Zmeskall (himself bed-ridden with severe gout). To Zmeskall he replied, "A thousand thanks for your sympathy. I do not despair. But what is most painful to me is the complete cessation of all my activities. Yet there is no evil which has not something good in it as well – May Heaven grant you too an alleviation of your painful condition. Perhaps we shall both be restored to health and then we shall meet and see one another again as friendly neighbors. Heartfelt greetings from your old friend who sympathizes with you."[212]

Beethoven's condition deteriorated progressively through March. He lost weight, became weaker, had difficulty focusing on and holding a steady conversation, sighed frequently, and perspired profusely. On 23 March, Schindler and Breuning assisted him with his final will, in which the whole of his estate was left to Karl and his "natural" heirs.[213] Late in March, he also made his peace with the church. His brother Johann, supported by Dr Wawruch, took the initiative and Beethoven acceded to the calling of a priest.[214] He then lay quietly lost in thought and amiably indicated by a nod his "I shall soon see you again." He received the last rites from a priest in the presence of Schindler, Breuning, Johann, and Johann's wife, Therese, who reported many years later that after receiving

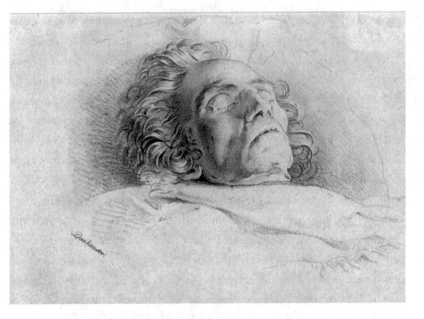

Beethoven on his death bed, March 1827. Based on a lithograph by
Josef Dannhausen. Beethoven-Haus, Bonn.

the viaticum, Beethoven said to the priest, "I thank you, ghostly sir! You
have brought me comfort." Shortly thereafter, likely on 23 or 24 March,
Beethoven uttered his well-known phrase, "Plaudite, amici, comoedia
finita est" (Applaud, friends, the comedy is finished).[215] A little later some
bottles of Mainz wine were brought to him and were placed on a table
beside his bed. He looked at them and murmured "Pity, pity – too late."[216]
These were his last words.

For the last three days of his life Beethoven was in a delirium, with only
rare moments of consciousness, likely the result of hepatic encephalopathy.[217] Schindler wrote, "The last days have been extraordinary; he antic-
ipates his death with true Socratic wisdom and great serenity of spirit."[218]
"At about one o'clock in the afternoon he showed the first signs of his
approaching death. A frightful struggle between death and life began,

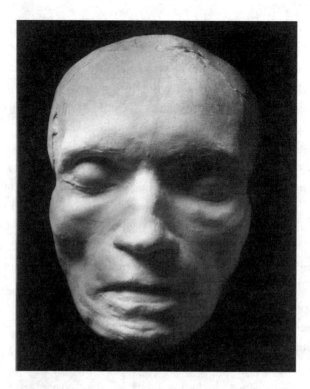

Death mask created shortly after Beethoven's death. Compare this mask with the life mask (fig. 11) created in 1812. Beethoven-Haus, Bonn.

probably as a result of his extraordinarily strong nervous system, and continued without respite until a quarter to six on March 26th when, during a heavy hailstorm, the great composer gave up his spirit."[219] Gerhard von Breuning confirms that a violent storm occurred at his death, Nature's eminently appropriate *son-et-lumière* salute.[220]

After Beethoven's death, his close friends, together with Johann, searched for the bank shares (Karl's inheritance), which eventually were found together with the letters to the "Immortal Beloved." The Heilegenstadt Testament was discovered six months later. Thayer lists Beethoven's valuables, furniture, and remaining possessions that were sold at an auction in November 1827, including a Broadwood piano, one cello, one viola, and two violins.[221] The list of fifty-three books sold at the auction provides a revealing glimpse of his wide-ranging interests: subjects include religion (7), travel (7), music (7), health (2), education (2), philosophy (1), a number of volumes of literature, history, and poetry, and a translation of Shakespeare's plays.[222]

The autopsy carried out the following day destroyed his features due to efforts to view his auditory apparatus. Many visitors – including "strangers," according to Gerhard von Breuning – also plucked locks of his hair as souvenirs; Breuning notes that not much hair was left by the time of the funeral, which took place three days after his death.[223] He also mentions "bed sores" found on his lower back. Such sores are often found in bed-bound individuals who have poor circulation and inadequate nursing care. Their presence was not mentioned in the autopsy report. The description of events in the room in the days following his death suggests that the scene was not an edifying one, to say the least.

The funeral was conducted from Trinity Church and thence to Währing Cemetery in a procession of an estimated 20,000 people, one of the largest ever in Vienna, including many notables. Among the musical works performed were the "Miserere" from the *Missa solemnis* and the funeral march from the Piano Sonata in A flat major, op. 26. Beethoven's remains were exhumed and reburied first in 1863 and again in 1888 when they were interred next to those of Franz Schubert in the Central Cemetery in Vienna.[224]

The funeral displayed the appreciation that Vienna had for its adopted composer-son. There had often been tensions between Beethoven and the music-loving Viennese public, and he sensed "enemies" among them whom he thought were out to denigrate, if not destroy him. But the city turned out in full force to honour his memory and his genius. He had arrived in Vienna thirty-five years previously, penniless and unknown. He had an eccentric character and medical problems that would have sunk a lesser mortal. Through creative genius and intense application he was able to rise above these hurdles and conquer not only Vienna, but the world. He had seized fate by the throat and it did not crush him.

CHAPTER THREE

Beethoven's Health Problems

For you, poor Beethoven, no happiness can come from outside. You must create everything for yourself in your own heart; and only in the world of ideas can you find friends.

Beethoven to Baron Ignaz von Gleichenstein
after rejection by Therese Malfatti[1]

Beethoven experienced a variety of health problems during his adult life and referred to them frequently in letters to family, friends, and business associates. His deafness is well-known, but most of his body systems were also affected at different times of his life. He refers most frequently to gastrointestinal and psychiatric symptoms in his correspondence, but respiratory, rheumatologic, and ophthalmologic symptoms also affected him intensely for shorter periods. We have five primary sources of information about Beethoven's health: his own letters, letters written by others, the Conversation Books, reports (including the autopsy report) written by his physicians, and a modern-day toxicological analysis of his hair.

BEETHOVEN'S LETTERS

Beethoven was an inveterate letter writer: at least 1,570 of his letters are extant. The earliest dates from 1787, when he was not yet seventeen, and his last letter was written in 1827, just a few days before his death. Many of these letters are addressed to business associates and publishers concerning his compositions. Others are to friends, family, and acquaintances. The first of two collections of Beethoven's letters in English translation, edited by J.S. Shedlock, was published in 1909.[2] A second collection, edited by Emily Anderson and published in 1961,[3] includes a number of letters that were unknown or unavailable at the time of the earlier publication. Anderson's work is widely cited and is the most accurate translation available at present. The material on which this chapter is based is derived largely from her translation.

Beethoven was not a master of language or grammar, and there are numerous errors in the original autographs.[4] A great majority of his letters are in German, but a few in French, addressed to correspondents in France, England, and Russia, also contain grammatical errors. However, the fact that Beethoven was not crafting his letters for posterity gives them an immediacy, spontaneity, and relevance that they might not otherwise possess: they reflect his state of mind and body at the time of writing. Since he was preoccupied with his health, and made references to health matters to most of his correspondents, his letters are a fertile source of medical information.

The analysis of this medical information given in the following tables was prepared by examining both the Shedlock and the Anderson translations and noting each reference to a symptom or a health-related problem, along with the nature, timing, and where possible the severity and duration: the result is a comprehensive chronological medical history based on Beethoven's self-reported symptoms. Any mention Beethoven made about "feeling better" was also noted as an indication of the duration of a symptom or an illness. All these results are summarized in six tables, so that the reader can follow the nature and the pattern of Beethoven's symptoms as they evolved over the years. For each symptom, the tables include the date, Beethoven's age at the time of writing, and the letter number from which the information was obtained. The symptoms are categorized according to the medical system affected: gastrointestinal (table 3.1), ear, nose, and throat (ENT; table 3.2), psychiatric and psycho-

TABLE 3.1   GASTROINTESTINAL SYMPTOMS

Date	Age	Letter	Symptoms
June 1801	30	51	"abdominal problems, colic and violent diarrhea"
Nov. 1805	34	124	"suffering colic pains – my usual complaint"
Feb. 1808	37	164	"attack of colic seized me yesterday"
Mar. 1808	37	165	"colic better"
Summer 1808	37	170	"wretched attack of colic"
Jan. 1810	39	244	"still suffering from my abdominal complaint"
May 1810	39	260	"have had a violent attack of colic – better today"
Sept. 1812	41	382	"Not well since yesterday – worse today. Caused by indigestible food."
Sept. 1814	43	493	"Health suffered a severe blow owing to inflammation of the intestines which brought me almost to death's door."
1816	45	729	"attack of colic to which I suddenly succumbed yesterday. Better today."
June 1818	47	904	"I fell very ill and will soon need something to restore my stomach."
1820	49	1041	"Sensitive abdomen. Need strong protecting belt."
July 1821	50	1054-5	attack of jaundice lasting six weeks
Nov. 1821	50	1059	violent diarrhea
July 1823	52	1219	feeling "very ill," "violent" diarrhea," stomach is "completely ruined"
Aug. 1823	52	1230	abdomen is still "thoroughly upset"
Apr. 1824	53	1276	sick from bad food
May 1825	54	1368 1370	convalescing from inflammation of intestines

continued on next page

somatic (table 3.3), respiratory (table 3.4), and ophthalmologic (table 3.5). All of Beethoven's references to "feeling better" are summarized in table 3.6. The following systems were either unaffected or minimally affected: central nervous, cardiovascular, musculoskeletal, genitourinary, and dermatological. One noteworthy finding from these tables is the frequent

TABLE 3.1 (CONT'D)

Date	Age	Letter	Symptoms
May 1825	54	1371	spits a "good deal of blood," but it is probably "only from my windpipe"[1] "I require stronger medicine but it must not be constipating."
May 1825	54	1373	suffering "a good deal" from diarrhea
May 1825	54	1382	stomach "not in order"
Aug. 1825	54	1416	stomach "in a bad state"
Aug.1825	54	1422	fresh and violent attack of abdominal trouble
Jan. 1827	56	1546	confined to bed with "dropsy"[2]

1 In the context of Beethoven's abdominal symptoms and the relative absence of respiratory problems in his final years, it is more likely that the blood originated in the gastrointestinal than in the respiratory tract.

2 ascites and liver failure (his final illness)

TABLE 3.2   ENT (EAR, NOSE, AND THROAT) SYMPTOMS

Date	Age	Letter	Symptoms
June 1801	30	51	hearing problem since three years ago, ears "hum and buzz day and night"
July 1801	30	53	"My most prized possession, my hearing, has greatly deteriorated." "It affects me most when in company, least when playing and composing."
Nov. 1801	30	54	humming and buzzing is slightly less especially in the left ear where the deafness began, hearing weaker
March 1809	38	205	"With my poor hearing I need someone always at hand."
Summer 1815	44	550	"Tormented by my poor hearing. I feel only <u>pain</u> in the society of others."
July 1817	46	790	poor hearing
Feb. 1822	51	1072	"Last night I succumbed to the earache which I usually suffer from during this season."
Sept. 1822	51	1101	"My poor hearing cuts me off to a certain extent from human society."
May 1825	54	1371	"Frequent nose bleeds which I often had last winter as well."

TABLE 3.3   PSYCHIATRIC AND PSYCHOSOMATIC SYMPTOMS

Date	Age	Letter	Symptoms
Sept. 1787	16	1	"Plagued with asthma,"[1] fears this will turn into consumption; also "melancholia" which is "almost as great a torture as my illness"
June 1801	30	51	now and then has a "raptus"[2]
Spring 1805	34	110	"private grief" (likely his hearing loss) "which has robbed me for a long time – of my usual energy"
June 1805	34	119	becoming more peevish every day
July 1809	38	220	"We have been suffering misery in concentrated form."
Dec. 1809	39	232	"Winter depresses me greatly – melancholy reminders."
Feb. 1810	39	250	poor "fitful" sleep, prefers wakefulness to any kind of sleep
Spring 1810	39	254	"Your news has again plunged me from the heights of the most sublime ecstasy down into the depths."[3]
May 1810	39	256	"I would have left this life long ago, what is more, by my own hand." (distress because of hearing loss)
Dec. 1812	42	394	"Since Sunday I have been ailing – mentally more than physically."
Jan. 1813	42	402	"moral factors" affecting health
May 1813	42	426	"A number of unfortunate incidents occurring one after the other have really driven me into a state bordering mental confusion." (likely financial difficulties)
Dec. 1813	43	441	"I am on the verge of despair."
Summer 1815	44	550	"peevish, sensitive, tormented" (by poor hearing) "I often feel only pain in the society of others."
Nov. 1815	44	571	"exhausted" because of "exertions" associated with death of brother

continued on next page

1 written shortly after the death of his mother from tuberculosis. Because there is no further reference to "asthma," it is likely that these were attacks of hyperventilation associated with his fears of contracting tuberculosis.

2 an episode of loss of control and absent-mindedness (see chapter 2, p. 34)

3 written after he was rejected in love by Therese Malfatti

TABLE 3.3   (CONT'D)

Date	Age	Letter	Symptoms
Feb. 1816	45	615	"My brother's death has affected my spirits and my nerves."
May 1816	45	633	"For the last six weeks I have been in very poor health, so much so that I have thought of my death."
1816	45	710	really ill, suffering from a nervous breakdown
1817	46	740	"I am angry, angry, angry."
July 1817	46	790	poor hearing and conflict with servants "drive me to despair"
Aug. 1817	46	805	"I often despair and would like to die … I can see no end to all my infirmities … if the present state of affairs does not cease next year I shall probably be in my grave."
1817	46	866	insomnia
1817	46	877	often thinks of death
July 1818	47	904	"heart attack" after conflict with nephew and with servants – likely chest wall pain associated with anxiety and frustration of situation
Jan. 1819	48	933	terrible event in family (nephew ran away to his mother), "For a time I was driven out of my mind."
June 1819	48	948	"despondency and several distressing circumstances" made him lose courage
July 1819	48	952	very unwell – worries about nephew
Sept. 1821	50	1056	difficulty sleeping, somnolence, dreaming
May 1822	51	1078	"I am very sensitive and irritable."
May 1825	54	1377	anger (toward nephew)
		1379	
June 1825	54	1387	conflict with nephew is having a bad effect on health
June 1826	55	1489	insomnia (anxiety re nephew)
Sept. 1826	55	1521	worn out and unhappy

association between illness and weather. Beethoven complained often and bitterly of the Viennese winters, and his health problems, both medical and psychiatric, were frequently worse in the winter and better in the summer months. This pattern is particularly clear in table 3.6: there are no reports of "feeling better" during winter months.

TABLE 3.4   RESPIRATORY SYMPTOMS

Date	Age	Letter	Symptoms
Spring 1805	34		"heavy cold"
Sept. 1813	42	430	has a cold
April 1814	43	473	heavy cold, feels very poorly, has to keep very quiet
May 1816[1]	45	632	"I have not been feeling well for a considerable time."
Nov. 1816	45	671	ill since October, eight days in bed, dangerous feverish cold
Dec. 1816	46	688	confined to room
Dec. 1816	46	712	state of health worse, "I have a heavy feverish cold."
Feb. 1817	46	758-9	feverish cold, very ill since 15 Oct.
Mar. 1817	46	771	15 Oct. succumbed to inflammatory fever, "from the effects of which I am still suffering and my art also."
Apr. 1817	46	776	"On 15 Oct., I contracted a serious illness."
Apr. 1817	46	779	"All this while I have not been very well."
June 1817	46	783	"I have developed a violent feverish cold."
July 1817	46	785	doctor diagnosed "disease of the lungs"
July 1817	46	788	feverish cold and disease of the lungs
July 1817	46	794	in poor health
July 1817	46	798	very ill yesterday
Sept. 1817	46	817	owing to a chill feels much worse
Dec. 1817	47	839	bad chill, cough, headache, cannot move
1817	47	854	feeling weaker
Jan. 1818	47	881 to 882	"pain so severe I had to lie on the couch," chill, violent cold and cough
Feb. 1818	47	892	"encore malade"
May 1818	47	900	last night again very ill
1818	47	921	cough
June 1819	48	948	in bed with violent cold
1819	48	995	another attack, stayed at home
		996	"I am a semi invalid."
		997	suffering from catarrh

continued on next page

1 The illnesses between mid-1816 and mid-1818 have been grouped together as "Respiratory" though the symptoms often were not specified. This seems appropriate because of his doctor's eventual diagnosis of "disease of the lungs" in July 1817. See text for further discussion.

TABLE 3.4 (CONT'D)

Date	Age	Letter	Symptoms
Aug. 1820	49	1032	took open chaise and caught cold
Aug. 1823	52	1230	caught catarrh and cold in head ("serious complaints for me") after traveling
Oct. 1825	54	1438	cold and catarrh
June 1826	55	1489	could not sleep because of coughing the whole night

TABLE 3.5 EYE SYMPTOMS

Date	Age	Letter	Symptoms
Apr. 1823	52	1167	not well, eye troubling him
May 1823	52	1180	eyes worse, "allow me to see everything, only very slowly"
May 1823	52	1182	sore eyes, three weeks, doctor forbids him to write or read
May 1823	52	1183	still has bad eye, but recovering
June 1823	52	1188	"If only eyes were cured, I could write again."
June 1823	52	1196	working as much as eyes allow
June 1823	52	1197	"My eyes must still be spared."
July 1823	52	1203	As yet cannot strain eyes for long, "my eyes bid me stop writing."
July 1823	52	1205	cannot stand town air because of eyes
July 1823	52	1207	disease of eyes for three months
	52	1208	eyes improving very slowly, "If only I did not wear glasses, would clear quickly."
July 1823	52	1214	eyes prevent him attending in person
July 1823	52	1215	town air has bad effect on eyes
Aug. 1823	52	1226	eye complaint 2½ months, not cured
Aug. 1823	52	1228	very ill, not only on account of eyes
Aug. 1823	52	1232	can now use eyes by daylight
Sept. 1823	52	1240	eye complaint rapidly clearing up
Jan. 1824	53	1260	still suffering from eye complaint

TABLE 3.6   HEALTH IMPROVED

Date	Age	Letter	Symptoms
Sept. 1807	36	151	health slowly improving
Autumn 1807	36	153	head beginning to feel better
Summer 1816	45	646	in excellent health
July 1817	46	792	health improving
Sept. 1817	46	820	health better
June 1818	47	903	health greatly improved
Sept. 1820	49	1033	health now completely restored
Nov. 1821	50	1061	health improving every day
May 1823	52	1183	at last recovering (from eye problems)
July 1823	52	1203	getting better now
July 1823	52	1208	eyes improving very slowly
July 1823	52	1210	health improving
July 1823	52	1215	"I am much better."
Sept. 1823	52	1240	health better

Several limitations of this procedure are apparent. First, Beethoven's comments about his health are often brief and general: examples include "I am unwell today," "Today I am ailing," "I have been in bed for a few days," or "I have a fever," with no further description of specific symptoms. References to symptoms or ill health in general rather than specific terms were assigned to the particular system that was the chief source of his complaints during that period of his life. For example, during the period 1816–19, he frequently experienced respiratory symptoms and rarely complained of symptoms derived from other systems; during these years, general health references have been categorized as respiratory system complaints.

Secondly, Beethoven uses terms that are no longer current in medical symptomatology, such as "catarrh" or "gout on the chest." A third difficulty is that the correspondence we have today is not complete: particularly in the early years, there are gaps of many months between extant letters, and we have no information on the state of his health in between.

A final problem is that not all his letters were dated clearly. In most instances Anderson was able to assign a year and possibly a month of an undated letter according to the content, context, or recipient; her dating system is followed throughout this chapter. In two letters that Anderson dates to 1814 with no month,[5] Beethoven states that he is "unwell, I dare not go out," and "Every other day I am ill, always ill." I believe these letters were likely written in the fall of 1814 because the only other clearly dated letter from 1814 in which he complains of medical problems is Anderson no. 493, dated September 1814; in this letter he describes inflammation of the intestines that had brought him "almost to death's door."

The references to his hearing are of great interest. While he rarely refers to his deafness in his letters, there is no doubt that it affected him deeply; when he does refer to his hearing loss, particularly in the early years, he describes it in strong language. There are no references to deafness in his correspondence for a period of almost eight years between July 1801 and March 1809,[6] and then for a further six years until the summer of 1815.[7] In comparison, during these same years there are frequent references to his gastrointestinal, psychological, and even, for a brief and later period, to eye problems. Could the relatively infrequent references to his hearing loss mean that his adaptation to this impairment was better than has been supposed?

As noted above, the central nervous, cardiovascular, musculoskeletal, genitourinary, and dermatological systems were either unaffected or minimally affected and were not included in the tables. In three letters he complains of headaches.[8] On six occasions he refers to problems related to the musculoskeletal system: in November 1810,[9] and October 1811[10] he mentions problems with his feet; in autumn 1817,[11] March 1821,[12] and February 1826[13] he complains of "rheumatism," which in 1821 lasted six weeks and is attributed to the "strange and terrible winter." In March 1808 he describes a "drastic nail operation" carried out because of a fingernail infection (paronychia).[14] Beethoven's only reference to gout is a statement that he has "gout on the chest,"[15] but two of his doctors refer to gout: in 1807, Dr Schmidt describes his headaches as "gout-related," and in 1826 Dr Braunhofer writes "Your dysentery is related to your gouty affliction.

You do not have rheumatism in your hands and your feet."[16] Despite these statements, it is unlikely that Beethoven had gout.

From November 1821 onward Beethoven made increasingly frequent references to his deteriorating health, particularly after November 1824. Also, in August–September 1821 he experienced a six-week episode of painless jaundice. Although he recovered, it is likely that his liver function was compromised for the final five and a half years of his life, and during this period he may have also suffered from undiagnosed conditions that commonly accompany liver disease, such as anaemia and malnutrition, which would explain at least some of his symptoms. It is interesting to note that at times Beethoven experienced emotional and physical symptoms concomitantly. For example, in his first letter, written in 1787 following the death of his mother,[17] he states he is plagued with "asthma" (or tightness around the chest; see chapter 2) and "melancholia," and that the latter was "almost as great a torture" as the former. In December 1812, he states "I have been ailing – mentally more than physically."[18]

Another feature is that Beethoven experienced gastrointestinal, psychiatric, and of course hearing problems either continuously or in a recurring fashion from the time of their onset to the end of his life, whereas the musculoskeletal, respiratory, and eye symptoms occurred in specific discrete time periods. The dates of the musculoskeletal symptoms are given above. With the exception of periodic "colds," the "asthma" following the death of his mother, and the probable pneumonia that sparked the onset of his final illness, his respiratory problems were wholly confined to the period from May 1816 to 1819. The eye problems occurred solely between April 1823 and January 1824. The "periodicity" exemplified by this analysis of his symptoms is of great assistance in determining the underlying cause(s).

LETTERS AND ACCOUNTS
WRITTEN BY OTHERS

On the whole, the letters written to or about Beethoven[19] are not helpful, but there are some exceptions. In a letter to Franz Wegeler of November

1804, Stephan von Breuning states that Beethoven's loss of hearing has had an "indescribable and bad" effect on him, and that "intercourse with him is a real exertion."[20] Breuning and Beethoven had lived in the same building from May until October of that year, and Breuning stated that shortly after they moved in together, Beethoven became "dangerously ill, followed by a prolonged fever." Since there is no other reference to an illness in mid-1804 it is difficult to determine the nature of this condition.

Beethoven attempted many remedies for his deafness. In 1805, he consulted a Father Weiss in Vienna, who had a special interest in deaf people and a reputation for achieving many cures.[21] Weiss instructed Beethoven to follow a specific diet, to rest, and to put as little strain on his ears as possible, but Beethoven was not able to persist in the treatment. There was no improvement in his condition. More than twenty years later he consulted Weiss again.[22] On this occasion, the treatment was a series of "oil injections" that Beethoven docilely accepted at first, but he stopped going after a few days and ignored a letter of warning from Weiss. Schindler ends this anecdote by noting Beethoven's "impatience and lack of respect for any medical treatment that did not achieve the hoped-for results within twenty-four hours."

Most other letters and reports are of a general nature and throw little light on medical issues. For example, in July 1825 Karl wrote to Peters, a music publishing firm, noting that his uncle's health was "severely impaired."[23] Later that year Tobias Haslinger comments to Johann Nepomuk Hummel that "Beethoven is aging very much" (he was fifty-five at the time).[24] Some letters refer to Beethoven's behavioural and emotional difficulties. Schindler describes "offensive" lawsuits, family troubles, and "base ingratitude" of friends that affected Beethoven's morale and caused "long periods of depression" after 1815.[25] Carl Czerny notes that Beethoven had worked so hard that his health had suffered, and he had developed hypochondria,[26] a statement with which Ignaz von Seyfried agrees and adds that the more Beethoven's hearing failed, and his intestinal troubles became worse, the more melancholic he became.[27] He increasingly perceived "delusion, malice and deceit" in those around him, and he became suspicious even of his closest friends. Wegeler also found Beethoven "suspicious by nature."[28] Friedrich Rochlitz notes that he was sometimes full of spontaneous merriment and other times seized by a profound melancholy.[29] L. Schlosser describes Beethoven's loss of temper and eccentric behaviour and justifies it on the basis of his hearing loss, isolation, and sensitive character.[30] Such letters confirm that Beethoven suffered from psychiatric problems that included hypochondria, melancholia, paranoid ideas about some of those around him, and eccentric behaviour.

THE CONVERSATION BOOKS

The Conversation Books are the writing pads that Beethoven's friends and visitors used to communicate with him from 1819 until his death in 1827. The complete set has been published in German,[31] but an English translation is not yet available. J.-G. Prod'homme translated portions of the text into French; this is the edition used for most of the references and quotations used in this book.[32] In his introduction, Prod'homme notes that Beethoven carried the books everywhere and that they contain discussions – albeit one-sided since Beethoven replied to the written comments verbally – on a wide variety of topics including politics, town gossip, literature, religion, children's education, history, philosophy, and "animal magnetism." Regrettably, we often have to guess at his replies. Prod'homme also notes that Schindler, who had possession of the books after Beethoven's death, destroyed or annotated some of the material, rendering it almost illegible. In this section I will present references made to Beethoven's health made by non-physicians. Those made by physicians, which are of special interest as some of the very few verbatim reports of doctor-to-patient communication we have from the pre-electronic era, will be reported in the following section.

In November 1819 Selig [a friend] states: "Mr Graff has a method of curing deafness and he would like to tell you about it. Take a black radish, rub it on cotton and then roll the cotton in your ear ... thanks to this simple technique, his wife regained her hearing in four weeks. At least it cannot do any harm."[33] On 5 January 1820, an unknown person, likely a sales agent, informs Beethoven that a neighbour, Wolfsohn, has developed three hearing aids, and invites Beethoven to go and try them out to see if they will help him; Wolfsohn claims that his hearing aid is visually subdued ("combiné optiquement").[34] Six weeks later, the following entries appear:

Beethoven: Wolfsohn is lying about me
Bernard [a friend]: In the paper one reads that you have used the Wolfsohn hearing aid with great success; it is placed like a diadem on the head and it is hidden by hair or by a wig. Must I complain on your behalf? [35]

In a footnote Prod'homme explains that an advertisement had appeared on 29 February in which Wolfsohn claimed to be a doctor of engineering. The advertisement claimed that the apparatus was fitted on to the heads of people with hearing difficulties, and that it was inconspicuous because it could simulate a lock of hair. Readers were assured that "our immortal Beethoven employed it with success." A correction published in the newspaper on 9 March announced that Beethoven had examined the hearing aid but had never used it.[36] From this anecdote we can infer that Wolfsohn had built the hearing aid and had tried without success to persuade Beethoven to use it, but nevertheless attempted to market it using Beethoven's name. He was "found out" by Beethoven and his friend and was persuaded to retract and correct his advertisement.

On 21 March 1820 Streicher (a friend) shows Beethoven two new ear trumpets made of wood. He states they fit the ear better than metal or brass. He then explains to Beethoven how he will connect an arc of wood to the piano; Beethoven is to apply it to his teeth or his skull to maximize the sound.[37]

There are no medical reports in Prod'homme's edition of the Conversation Books for 1821 and part of 1822, and Prod'homme alleges that Schindler destroyed the papers for this period.[38] This paucity of information is regrettable because we know from Beethoven himself that in August 1821 he experienced an episode of jaundice. Entries made by physicians who visited during this illness would be helpful in making diagnostic inferences. Schindler erroneously describes Beethoven as enjoying good health in 1821[39] and makes no reference to the attack of jaundice; it is inconceivable that Schindler was not aware of it, not only because he was working as Beethoven's secretary by this time, but he also had access to Beethoven's correspondence and the Conversation Books when he wrote his biography of Beethoven. We can only conclude that Schindler destroyed them because they contained information about Beethoven that was inconsistent with the portrait of the composer he wished to draw.

On 16 January 1823 Johann (Beethoven's brother, who is an apothecary) asks, "Do you still have colic?" Beethoven must have replied yes, for Johann goes on: "You should take some rhubarb powder, follow a good diet, avoid fish altogether, and drink lots of water."[40] In mid-April there is a discussion between Sandra (a man who is deaf) and Beethoven, both communicating in writing. Beethoven describes the treatments, particularly baths and country air, that have helped, and adds, "Do not start using hearing aids too soon. By abstaining I have retained my left ear a little ... lately I have not been able to stand galvanism. It is sad: doctors do not know much; one tires of them eventually."[41]

In late April 1823 Beethoven complains of pain in his eyes. Schupanzigh (a violinist friend) replies, "Do not wash your eyes with water. Rheumatism of the eyes is less serious than leucorrhoea; the clear and pure air of the country will cure all your troubles."[42] The following July Stein and Haslinger (publishers) introduce Beethoven to a visitor from Leipzig who is a specialist in homeopathic medicine. They refer to Hahnemann (the founder of homeopathy) and the visitor states: "They gave examples of people who had even more severe deafness than you, and who got fixed up in four to six weeks using a simple and non-painful technique ... the treatment is a *natural* method."[43] In Baden that summer Beethoven (addressing Schindler) writes: "My doctor saved me, because I could no longer write music, but now I can write notes which help relieve me of my troubles." Here Beethoven was likely referring to an eye problem that he had had for several months and that had interfered with his ability to compose.[44] In August 1823 Karl (Beethoven's nephew) recommends homeopathic medicine for Beethoven's deafness. "Homeopathy is now fashionable. Dr Braunhofer prescribed homeopathic doses because he follows fashions in medicine."[45]

These interactions between Beethoven and his visitors from the Conversation Books illustrate the large number of herbal, pharmacological, electrical, and mechanical techniques used in the eternally hopeful attempt to treat his deafness.

PHYSICIANS' REPORTS

Ordinarily, the reports of Beethoven's physicians would have been a key source of information about his medical problems. It is not known to what extent his physicians kept personal medical records about Beethoven, as none of these notes has yet come to light. However, we do have letters written by physicians and the Conversation Books constitute another valuable source, although there are not many instances of interactions with physicians until his final illness. The most complete medical report available is that by Andreas Wawruch, Beethoven's physician during his final illness, written just six weeks after the composer's death. This report is paraphrased in the discussion on Wawruch below; the full text is given in Appendix 4.

Beethoven was treated by at least eleven physicians during his lifetime.[46] The following account presents a brief biographical sketch of each one (in the approximate chronological order in which they cared for him), together with what is known of the treatments they utilized.[47] Most were illustrious medical men in Vienna and some had reputations throughout Europe. One must question the opinions of Schindler,[48] Gerhard von Breuning,[49] and others who have harshly criticized the medical treatment that Beethoven received. It was poor by our standards, but it was the best that could be offered in Vienna, or in the world, during that period. The limitations of the treatments to which he was subjected were due not to the modest skills of his physicians but to the limitations in medical knowledge of the period.

Johann Peter Frank (1745–1821) was appointed director of the General Hospital in Vienna in 1795, and subsequently became a professor of medicine at the University of Vienna and a physician to the Austrian army. In 1809 Napoleon invited him to take a position in Paris, but he refused. Frank was a progressive thinker, and in 1786 he published an influential book on public health that became a standard text; in it he describes how governments can act to improve the health of their citizens.[50]

Frank was one of Beethoven's physicians between 1801 and 1809. In a letter of 1801 to Franz Wegeler, Beethoven refers to Frank disparagingly and describes his health problems, stating that his hearing loss was:

supposed to have been caused by the condition of my abdomen which, as you know, was wretched even before I left Bonn, but has become worse in Vienna where I have been constantly afflicted by diarrhea and have been suffering in consequence from extraordinary debility. Frank tried to tone up my constitution with strengthening medicines, and my hearing with almond oil, but much good did it do me! His treatment had no effect, my deafness became even worse, and my abdomen continued in the same state as before. Such was my condition until the autumn of last year; and sometimes I gave way to despair. [51]

There is little further information about Frank's treatments and it is not known why he ceased to be Beethoven's physician.

Johann Schmidt (1759–1809) was an army surgeon and a professor of anatomy at the University of Vienna. He had a special interest in ophthalmology and developed an international reputation through his writings. From 1801 until his death in 1809 Schmidt was Beethoven's physician. In a letter to Wegeler of November 1801, Beethoven asks: "What is your opinion of Schmidt? It is true that I am not inclined to change doctors ... Schmidt is a totally different fellow and, what is more, he might perhaps not be so casual – people talk about miraculous cures by galvanism; what is your opinion? A medical man told me in Berlin he saw a deaf and dumb child recover its hearing and a man who had also been deaf for seven years recover his."[52] Beethoven's hope that Schmidt might not be so "casual" is likely an implied criticism of Johann Frank, his physician at the time. In the Heiligenstadt Testament (see chapter 2), after describing his distress resulting from his hearing loss, Beethoven appeals: "When I am dead, request on my behalf Professor Schmidt, if he is still living, to describe my disease, and attach this written document to his record, so that after my death at any rate, the world and I may be reconciled as far as possible."

Schmidt and his family were interested in music. In January 1805 Beethoven wrote a letter in French to Dr Schmidt, dedicating the String Quartet in F major, op. 18, no. 1, to him:

I know well that the celebrity of your name, and the friendship with which you honour me, require that I dedicate this important work to you. The main reason why I decided to offer you this dedication is that the piece is more easily played, and can be enjoyed in the friendly circle of your family. In addition, once the excellent talents of your dear daughter have been developed, we will see that this aim will be met. I shall be happy with the result. This is an inadequate sign of my high esteem, and of my gratitude to you. I extend to you my very real and cordial sentiments.[53]

Two and a half years later, during the summer of 1807, Beethoven must have had an episode of illness, although he made no reference to it in his own correspondence. On 22 July 1807 Dr Schmidt wrote to Beethoven:

I was, dear friend, previously convinced that your headache was gout-related [*gichtisch*], and I am, now that the tooth has been pulled, still convinced of it. Your suffering will be reduced but it will not totally disappear, in Baden or even in Robaun, because the cold North wind [*Boreas*] is your enemy. Therefore leave Baden now, or if you want to try Robaun for eight days, go there right away, in order to put laurel [*Seitelbast*] bark on your arms. From leeches we can expect no further relief, but we can expect improvement if you walk briskly, work less, and sleep, as well as eating well, and drinking moderate amounts of alcoholic beverages. [54]

From this letter we learn that Beethoven had problems with his teeth and that his headache was thought to be "gout-related." We also learn that he had leeches applied, although it is not clear whether they were for his headache or for another unspecified medical complaint. It is possible that the leeches were used to treat his deafness, since various forms of blood letting were a recognized treatment for deafness at that time. It is reasonable to infer that Beethoven was treated by blood letting at some point in his life, but this letter is the only documentation we have. It is curious that Beethoven appears never to have mentioned bleeding in any of his correspondence. Perhaps, for some reason, it embarrassed him. The mention of gout suggests that he may also have had rheumatologic symptoms such as muscle and joint pain. Beethoven must have taken Schmidt's advice that he leave Baden immediately, because shortly thereafter, in a letter from Baden addressed to Baron von Gliechenstein, he writes: "After Schmidt's diagnosis, I must not stay here any longer."[55] There is no further mention of Schmidt in any correspondence, and the doctor died two years later in 1809.

Gerhard von Vering (1755–1823) was a military surgeon and a physician in the General Hospital in Vienna. He had studied in both France and England and became well known as a dermatologist and an otologist. He was the first physician Beethoven consulted about his deafness. In a letter to Wegeler of November 1801, Beethoven states:

For the last few months Vering has made me apply to both arms <u>vesicatories</u> which, as you doubtless know, consists of a certain kind of bark. Well, it is an extremely unpleasant treatment, inasmuch as for a few days (until the bark has drawn sufficiently) I am always deprived of the free use of my arms, not to mention the pain I have to suffer. True enough, I cannot deny it, the humming and buzzing is slightly less than it used to be, particularly in my left ear, where my deafness really began. But so far my hearing is certainly not a bit better; and I am inclined to think, although I do not dare to say so definitely, that it is a little weaker – The condition of my abdomen is improving, and especially when I have taken tepid baths for a few days I feel pretty well for eight or even ten days afterwards. I very rarely take a tonic for my stomach and, if so, only one dose. But following your advice I am now beginning to apply <u>herbs to my belly</u> – Vering won't hear of me taking shower baths. On the whole I am not at all satisfied with him. He takes far too little interest in and trouble with a complaint of this kind. I should never see him unless I went to his house, which is very inconvenient for me ... Vering is too much of a practitioner to derive many new ideas from reading.[56]

Beethoven must have conveyed his disgruntlement about these treatments to the doctor, because von Vering did not remain Beethoven's physician for much longer.

Andreas Bertolini was an assistant to Giovanni Malfatti (see below) and was Beethoven's physician and friend between 1809 and 1816. Little is known about Dr Bertolini and his treatment of Beethoven. In 1831, four years after Beethoven's death, he developed cholera and, believing himself to be dying, ordered all of his reports and letters about Beethoven to be destroyed;[57] he did not, in fact, die but lived into his nineties. Thayer interviewed him for the biography of Beethoven and includes information from Bertolini about Beethoven's music but not about Beethoven's medical problems.[58] This did not stop Newman from alleging that Bertolini had told Thayer that Beethoven suffered from syphilis, a detail that Thayer chose to exclude from the publication.[59]

Giovanni Malfatti (1774–1859) was born in Tuscany, completed his medical studies in Bologna, and moved to Vienna in 1795 to work with Johann Frank. Although he was a private practitioner, he became well known as the author of *Entwerf einer Pathogenie* (An Outline of Pathogenesis, 1809). He became Beethoven's physician in 1808, and he remained in this position with the help of his assistant Dr Bertolini until he and Beethoven quarrelled and parted ways in 1816. In 1801 Beethoven had proposed marriage to Dr Malfatti's niece, Therese Malfatti (see chapter 2). According to Malfatti's description Beethoven was "a disorderly (*konfuser*) fellow – but all the same he may be the greatest genius."[60] In 1811, when Beethoven was suffering from headaches, Malfatti recommended the waters of Teplitz, to which Beethoven acceded. A year later, Beethoven returned to Teplitz, and it was on this occasion that he met Goethe.

After their breakup, Beethoven had little to do with Dr Malfatti until his final illness, when Schindler, believing then that Malfatti would provide better treatment for the mortally ill composer, made strenuous efforts to effect a reconciliation between Malfatti and Beethoven. On 19 January 1827, three months before Beethoven's death, Schindler wrote to Beethoven, and after explaining that he had set up an appointment for Malfatti to visit Beethoven in Wawruch's absence, states: "What I am asking you, however, is to make a complete reconciliation with him concerning the past for it still rankles with him to a certain extent; only today he again gave me to understand that he could not forget this planned offense as he called it – some words of explanation from you will get everything to rights, and bring it back on the old friendly track."[61] Malfatti did visit and was reconciled with Beethoven. He recommended frozen fruit punch (which contained some alcohol) with excellent initial results. However, he declined to become more involved in the daily management of Beethoven's care, which was left in the hands of Dr Wawruch. As a result of Malfatti's treatment, Beethoven's spirits, if not his physical condition, improved so much that a month later Beethoven wrote to Schindler: "Truly a miracle ++. Those very learned gentlemen [presumably Wawruch and Seibert] have both been beaten; and it is only thanks to Malfatti's skill that my life is being saved."[62] Alas, the improvement was temporary; he died less than two weeks later.

Jakob von Staudenheim (1764–1830) completed medical studies in Paris before moving to Vienna, where he set up in private practice. He became well known as physician to members of the imperial family. He attended Beethoven occasionally before he became the composer's regular physician in 1817 and was a strong supporter of Beethoven's "cures" at Baden and other health spas.

Beethoven refers to Staudenheim a number of times in his correspondence. In 1812, writing to the publishers Breitkopf and Härtel in Leipzig, he states: "My Aesculapius [Dr Staudenheim] has led me round and round in a circle, seeing that after all the best cure is to be found in Teplitz. Those fellows have a poor idea of producing an effect; and I consider that in that respect we composers have undoubtedly outstripped them in our art."[63] In a letter to Frau Nanette Streicher of 1816, when Beethoven was suffering from a number of symptoms and health problems, he writes: "Furthermore, I may never be cured. I myself am inclined to distrust my present doctor who has finally pronounced my condition to be caused by <u>disease of the lungs</u>."[64] A year later, still very symptomatic, he writes: "My doctor [Staudenheim] thinks that to travel would be very good for my health."[65] A letter to Archduke Rudolf of 1819 states, "Meanwhile I have been in town a few times to consult my doctor – the persistent worries connected with my nephew who has been morally almost ruined are largely the cause of my indisposition."[66] To Franz Brentano in 1821 he writes: "During the whole summer I was suffering from jaundice, a complaint which persisted until the end of August. On Staudenheim's orders I had also to betake myself in September to Baden ... the weather soon became chilly, and I started such violent diarrhea that I could not stand the cure and had to rush back to Vienna."[67]

A letter to his brother Johann of May 1822 states: "On Staudenheim's orders I must still continue to take medicine and must not move about too much."[68] In August, again to Johann, he writes "Staudenheim absolutely insists on my going to Baden."[69] A third letter to his brother, written in September, states "The additional work is very difficult to fit in with my water and bath cures, the more so as Staudenheim has now advised me to bathe for an hour and a half."[70] Thayer reports that Staudenheim had insisted on strict obedience to his prescriptions.[71] Because Beethoven was unsuccessful in his efforts to get Dr Staudenheim to make a home visit, Staudenheim was no longer involved in his care after 1825, and he declined to attend Beethoven in his final illness, other than briefly as a consultant.

Carl Smetana (1774–1827) was a well-known Viennese surgeon with an interest in ophthalmology and otology. In 1816 he had carried out a successful operation for repair of a hernia on Beethoven's nephew Karl. In 1822, Beethoven consulted Smetana about his deafness. Smetana prescribed medication to be taken internally, from which Beethoven inferred that the doctor did not expect much improvement.[72] The dosage apparently read: "One teaspoon to be taken every hour," but Schindler reports Beethoven saying, "Bah, what good is a mere teaspoonful – it ought to say a tablespoonful ... So the bottle was empty in a few hours and the prescription must be refilled. The patient's progress is poor, the patient feels much worse than before starting the treatment for he is forced to drink large quantities of water, thereby precluding the slightest chance of any benefit from the medicine." Beethoven clearly had serious problems complying with medical advice. Beethoven also consulted Smetana about his eye problems in 1823. In a letter to Schindler he states, "I have to bandage my eyes at night, and must spare them a good deal, for, if I don't, as Smetana writes, I shall write very few more notes."[73] In 1825 Beethoven consulted him for a stomach problem.[74] Then, after Karl's suicide attempt in 1826, Beethoven wrote a desperate letter to Smetana, appealing for help in treating Karl,[75] but by the time Smetana received the letter, another surgeon was already involved in the case.

Beethoven had periodically consulted with Dr Anton Braunhofer (birth and death dates unknown) after 1820,[76] and in April 1825 wrote the following letter to him: "My Esteemed Friend, I am not feeling well and I hope that you will not refuse to come to my help, for I am in great pain. If you can possibly visit me today, I do most earnestly beg you to come – In constant gratitude and with my best regards, your Beethoven."[77] Braunhofer did come, and a month later Beethoven wrote a letter of appreciation: "Most Excellent and Amazingly Intelligent Sir, We thank you for the advice which was well given and well followed by means of the wheels of your inventive genius; and we inform you that in consequence we now feel very well. Our heart and soul are inclined to overflow and might therefore cause you, Sir, some inconvenience. Hence we are observing a reverend silence. Beethoven."[78]

A month later, Beethoven paid a visit to Dr Braunhofer's home and finding him not in left a canon (see the full description of this communication in chapter 1). Braunhofer's visit to Beethoven in April 1825 is recorded in the Conversation Books:

Dr B: No wine, no coffee, no spices. I will speak with your cook.

I guarantee you then a perfect recovery. I am sure you understand that this is important to me as your admirer and your friend.

An illness does not disappear in one day.

I will not bother you any longer with medicines; but only prescribe the diet, which will not make you die of hunger.

Your fever will have a short duration, yours is coming down already.

Karl: Yours is an inflammatory fever for which there is no agreeable remedy. Dr Staudenheimer (sic) also banned all wines.

Dr B: You must keep yourself occupied during the day *in order to be able to sleep at night*. If you want to feel well and live a long life, you must live in conformity with nature. You have a substantial predisposition to inflammation and it does not require much for you to have a serious intestinal inflammation. The cause is still in your body.

I will give you a powder.

I bet then if you take alcohol, you will become weak and faint within a few hours.

You would be a second Brown if you had studied medicine.

Facsimile of a letter of 11 July 1825 from Beethoven to Dr Braunhofer requesting an appointment. Collection H.C. Bodmer. Beethoven-Haus, Bonn.

Once you have been at Baden for a while you will feel better … When are you leaving?
Don't forget the music which you promised me. Just a few notes. I wish only to have an autograph from you. [Beethoven obliged a month later from Baden.]
You will be helped by fresh air. Walks are too tiring.
In the country you will enjoy fresh milk.[79]

The above is a fascinating example of a doctor-patient interaction. Much of Braunhofer's advice is sound common sense – be patient, work with nature, sleep well, enjoy fresh air, eat nourishing food, avoid alcohol – but the doctor also emphasizes his expertise and his authority; surprisingly, he does not offer Beethoven any medication. He provides his patient with a medical diagnosis – intestinal inflammation – and states that the patient has a "substantial predisposition" to it. Finally, the doctor gently reminds Beethoven about the need for payment for his services in the form of a short, autographed, musical composition.

To Schindler in August 1825 while in Baden, likely in reference to an eye problem that had been troubling him for the previous nine months, Beethoven writes : "My doctor saved me, because I could no longer write music, but now I can write notes which help to relieve me of my troubles."[80] The Conversation Books also contain comments by his nephew Karl, who writes that homeopathic medicine is now fashionable and he recommends it for Beethoven's hearing problem. He states that Dr Braunhofer prescribed homeopathic doses for Beethoven because he too follows fashions in medicine. On 23 February 1826 Dr Braunhofer writes,

If you want to get better quickly you must follow the diet that I prescribed for you last year, otherwise I cannot predict how long it will last.
No wine, no kaffeh (sic). Follow the diet and otherwise you can have as much as you want.
For a few days at least drink the best water you can get, and also almond milk.
Your dysentery is related to your gouty affliction. You do not have rheumatism in the hands nor the feet. No dizziness? Bitter taste? Heart palpitations? Humming in the ears?

Two or three times a day you must syringe yourself with warm milk. Cream of rice and cream of cereal will do you much good. When I leave I will give your woman servant a chocalate [sic] and if you give me two florins I will buy you a book and your servant can come and fetch it at my place.

I have to emphasize the importance of abstaining from wine for a few days and let you know your news. After tomorrow I hope that improvement will begin.

Place a flannel on your back as frequently as possible.

I reply that it is only by this means that you will get back your health quickly and avoid the noxious effects of the drugs.

The vial contains only water with one drop. You must drink it down and then be patient if tomorrow you are not quite well.

Dr Braunhofer: Kaffeh [sic] in any case, has a noxious effect on the lower stomach and on the whole organism. [Beethoven no doubt replies to each of the questions or comments put to him by Dr Braunhofer.]

Kaffeh augments and exaggerates the activity of the nerves, and this is its drawback for you. I will give you another prescription today.

How much powder do you still have?

Let me know in two days how it's going and I will give you another remedy.

Stimulants relieve for a while, but subsequently have a bad effect.

I am going to give you a stimulant (quinchina) but only a very small dose. This will certainly help you if you follow the diet that I have given you.[81]

In these instructions, Dr Braunhofer again emphasizes the importance of diet, avoidance of alcohol and stimulants (coffee), drinking plenty of fluids (water), and a warm flannel for its soothing effect. On this occasion, he prescribes a small dose of medication (quinchina). Beethoven continued to consult Dr Braunhofer until February 1826, when he wrote the following letter to him.

Esteemed Friend! I am extremely obliged to you for your attentive care for my health. So far as it has been possible, I have kept to your prescriptions; of wine, coffee and everything else I have drunk only the amounts you ordered. It is difficult to judge at once the extent of the effect of your treatment after only a few days. The pain in my back is not severe, I admit, but it shows that the trouble is still there. So that I believe that I am right in using the medicines you sent me today (but I don't know how much they cost) – Don't neglect your own welfare when attending to the health of other people. I am extremely sorry not to be able to prescribe something for you in return and must leave you to your own devices – I hope to see you as soon as possible – With kindest regards, your grateful Beethoven.[82]

On Beethoven's return to Vienna in December 1826 at the onset of his final illness, Dr Braunhofer declined to attend to Beethoven, ostensibly because of distance to the composer's home would make frequent calls difficult. However, one wonders if he was offended by Beethoven's well-meaning but clumsy and possibly patronizing comments in the above letter.

Andreas Wawruch (1773–1842) was a well-known medical teacher and physician in Vienna, who had published widely in the field of infections and parasitic diseases. He was also an accomplished musician with an admiration for Beethoven's music. He became Beethoven's physician fortuitously on 5 December 1826 and attended the composer until his death.[83] Wawruch's involvement came about in part because Staudenheim, Malfatti, and Braunhofer had refused to attend Beethoven, although Staudenheim and Malfatti did see him on a consultative basis during his final months. Seven weeks after Beethoven's death Wawruch published a detailed report on the composer's health problems and terminal illness.[84] This report describes Beethoven as having a "rugged" constitution. From the age of thirty he had suffered from both hearing loss and intestinal problems. The hearing loss was initially accompanied by "roaring and buzzing," and the intestinal problems by hemorrhoids, belching, and alternating constipation and diarrhea. Wawruch notes that Beethoven had developed a liking for "spirituous liquors ... with excessive use of strong punch," and seven years earlier this had caused a near mortal illness; subsequently, it gave rise to intestinal pain and colic, swollen feet, and the eventual development of his fatal illness, which began when on his return to Vienna from the country early in December. During a "cold and frosty night" he stopped at a village inn that lacked heat and winter windows.

Beethoven became feverish, was thirsty, and developed pains in his side. When Dr Wawruch first saw him, two days after his return to Vienna, he had inflammation of the lungs, was coughing blood, and had difficulty breathing. His pain was relieved by lying on his back. By the seventh day his condition had improved, but the following day he became jaundiced, developed vomiting and diarrhea, and was writhing with abdominal pain. As the ankle swelling, jaundice, and dropsy became much worse, with the agreement of Dr Staudenheim, an abdominal puncture was performed by the surgeon Dr Johann Seibert, and a large volume of fluid was released. Although the wound became infected, Beethoven's condition seemed to respond to this treatment; three subsequent punctures, all performed by Dr Seibert, were without complications. Beethoven refused to take any medications other than "gentle laxatives," and gradually lost his appetite and his strength. After consulting with Dr Malfatti "who was aware of Beethoven's inclination for spirituous liquors," iced punch and wine were recommended, which brought a temporary improvement in his condition. Unfortunately Beethoven abused the prescription, grew stuporose as if intoxicated, and had to be deprived of this "valuable stimulant." As the end approached, Dr Wawruch advised Beethoven that a priest be called, to which the composer agreed "with pious resignation." A few hours later, he lost consciousness, became comatose, and breathed with a "rattle." He died at about six in the afternoon, during a storm in which there was snow, thunder, and lightning.

Wawruch's report represents the most detailed description we have of Beethoven's medical problems from a physician's perspective. The report opens with a brief overview of Beethoven's health and character before meeting Wawruch, provides a detailed description of his final illness, and ends with the drama of his final days and death. Wawruch's use of non-technical language indicates that he was directing this report to a wider lay public rather than a medical audience. It is also clear from this account that Wawruch considered that Beethoven had an alcohol problem and notes that Malfatti, who had known the composer for a much longer period, agreed on this point. Wawruch seems to relate Beethoven's liver problems and "dropsy" to the alcohol.

Both Schindler and Gerhard von Breuning are highly critical of Wawruch's opinion that Beethoven abused alcohol,[85] but, as noted in chapter 2, Schindler qualified his opinion by conceding that during 1825–26 Beethoven drank to excess at times under the influence of Karl Holz. Elsewhere Schindler agrees that Beethoven "enjoyed" wine and fortified wine.[86] Gerhard von Breuning was only thirteen at the time of Beethoven's death, and although he clearly was a mature and articulate child, he could not have known much about Beethoven's past health and behaviour. By the time he wrote his biography of Beethoven, he was in his sixties and likely was reflecting the prevailing myths about Beethoven's drinking habits that had been carefully nurtured by Schindler and others.

Dr Wawruch's treatment during Beethoven's terminal illness, with the support of Drs Malfatti, Staudenheim, and Seibert, was only palliative. Given what we now know about Beethoven's underlying disease process, this is the only approach that was likely to be efficacious. Symptom relief is the key objective of present-day palliative care, and it is noteworthy that the alcohol recommended by Dr Malfatti relieved Beethoven's symptoms. In the context of current palliative treatment guidelines, it was not appropriate for Dr Wawruch to stop Beethoven's alcohol during the final weeks of his life.

THE AUTOPSY

Dr Johann Wagner, the last physician to deal with Beethoven, was the pathologist who conducted the autopsy, the day after Beethoven's death. Wagner wrote his report in Latin. Several English or French translations have been published, but none is entirely satisfactory; the most accurate is that by J.P. Horan.[87] The remaining renditions are difficult to interpret because the translations are too literal, the anatomical structures are hard to identify, and on occasion the translation is plainly inaccurate. Even the version in Thayer's biography of Beethoven contains mistranslations, possibly because the report was translated from a German version rather than the original Latin.[88] For these reasons, I have provided a new translation of the original report.[89] I have divided the report into paragraphs

Protocollum.
de sectione corporis Domini Ludwig van Beethoven.

Corpus mortui imprimis in extremitatibus valde tabe-
-factum ac petechiis nigris conspersum, abdomen nimis hydro-
-pice tumefactum contentumque. Cartilago auris magna et
irregulariter formata conspecta est, fossa scaphoidea
praeprimis vero concha eiusdem amplissima atque di-
-midio altior solito erat; anguli diversi et sulci ad-
-modum elevati erant. Meatus acusticus externus imprimis
ad membranam tympani occultam squamis cutis niten-
-tibus obsessus apparuit. Tuba Eustachii valde incrassata
eius membrana mucosa evasa ac ad partem osseam
paululum angustata erat. Cellulae conspicuae processus
mastoidei magni qui incisura non insignitus, membrana
mucosa sanguinolenta obvelatae erant. Ubertatem sangu-
-inis similem substantia cuncta ramis vasorum conspi-
-cuis paterta ossis petrosi, imprimis regione cochleae,
eius membrana spiralis paulum rubefacta conspecta,
aeque demonstravit. Nervi faciei valde incrassati erant.
Nervi acustici e contrario corrugati et sine medulla
erant. Arteriae auditivae iuxta eos decurrentes ultra
lumen culmi corvini dilatatae et cartilaginosae erant.
Nervus acusticus sinister multo tenuior cum teibus lineis
albidis tenuissimis, dexter cum crassiori candida linea e
substantia multo consistentiori et sanguine abundantiori
in hoc ambitu ventriculi quarti orti sunt. Sulci ceterum
multo mollioris et aquatici cerebri, altero tanto profundi
ac (ampliores) numerosiores quam solito visi sunt.
Calvarium et integro validam densitatem et crassitudinem
fere dimidium pollicis metiens obtulit. Cavum
thoracis itemque eius viscera indolem normalem
demonstravit. Cavum abdominis quatuor mensuris
albide fungiosi liquoris repletum erat. Hepar in
dimidium sui voluminis redactum corio simile, densa
colore subviridiescentes conspicatum et in sua

*Photocopy of the autopsy report for Beethoven. The original is held at the
Anatomisches-Pathologische Staadts Museum in Vienna.*

with subheadings (the original was written in one dense paragraph), but
this structure does not change the sequence of the text. A few liberties
were taken in rendering the original into modern English, but I believe
the accuracy has been retained. The objective was to make a translation
of the report that was comprehensible and easy to read. The diagnostic
implications of this autopsy report are discussed in chapter 4.

General Appearance

The body of the deceased was emaciated, and the skin was dotted with
black petechiae especially at the extremities; the abdomen was swollen
and the skin was stretched because of fluid in the abdominal cavity.

The External Ear

The aural cartilage appeared large and was of irregular shape; the fossae of the helix (scapha) and the concha were larger and deeper than usual by about one half. The crura and notches were more prominent than usual. Shiny scales of skin lined the external auditory canal, especially around the tympanic membrane, which they concealed.

The Middle and Internal Ear

The Eustachian tube was thickened, and its mucus membrane was swollen, but it became shrunken near its bony section. The mastoid process was sectioned and a vascular membrane lined the cellular structures within. Similarly, the petrous bone was covered by many blood vessels, especially towards the cochlea. The membranous part of the spiral lamina of the cochlea appeared redder than usual.

Both facial nerves were thickened. On the other hand, the two auditory nerves were wrinkled and lacked a central core. The auricular arteries encircled the auditory nerves, and were larger in size than a crow's feather. They also were cartilaginous. The left auditory nerve was much thinner than the right nerve, and had three dull white streaks on its surface; the right auditory nerve had a thick white streak of a substance having a dense consistency. It was vascularized as it curved around the floor of the fourth ventricle.

Brain and Cranium

The convolutions of the brain were softer and moister, and appeared to be deeper and more numerous than usual. In general, the bones of the cranium showed increased density and were almost one half inch thick.

The Thorax

The thoracic cavity, and the organs it contained, appeared normal.

The Abdomen

The abdominal cavity was filled with four quarts ["measures"] of a reddish, cloudy fluid. The liver was half of its usual size. It was compact and leathery in consistency, blue-green in color, and its surface was covered by nodules the size of a bean. Its vessels were very narrow and thickened and there was no blood in them. The gall bladder contained a dark colored fluid, and much gravel-like sediment.

The spleen appeared twice its usual size, and was compact and black in color. The pancreas also appeared larger and more compact, and the end of the pancreatic duct was the width of a goose feather. The stomach and the intestines were both distended with air. Both kidneys were pale red and soft in consistency. They were covered by cellular tissue about one inch in thickness, and this tissue was filled with a dark cloudy fluid. In each calyx there was a calcareous concretion approximately the size of half a pea.

A HAIR ANALYSIS

In 1996 a toxicological analysis was carried out on a lock of Beethoven's hair. Russell Martin has described the origin and epic wanderings of this hair sample, taken shortly after he died.[90] The lock of hair was finally acquired by a group of American investigators, who arranged for a chemical analysis of a few strands.[91] The analysis indicated that the hair did not contain opiate derivatives, mercury or arsenic, a finding that is consistent with Wawruch's report that Beethoven refused most medications during his final illness. However, it also revealed an average of sixty parts per million of lead, which is a hundred times more than the North American average. The authors conclude that Beethoven had "plumbism" (lead poisoning) and that this had contributed to his death. They speculated that the lead could have originated from the mineral water Beethoven consumed at spas, and/or from dishes or wine stored in lead-lined flasks or crystal. Another possible source of this lead is discussed in chapter 4.

The description of Beethoven's medical symptoms and problems presented in this chapter has been put together using only information derived from primary sources. This description demonstrates that the composer suffered not only from deafness but also from illnesses affecting his gastrointestinal, respiratory, ophthalmic, and musculoskeletal systems, and that he had psychiatric problems. A summary of his medical history in the format of a case conference is given in Appendix 2.

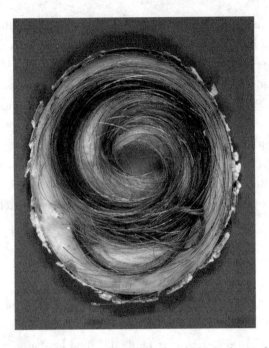

The Guevara lock of Beethoven's hair; an analysis of several hairs
from this lock showed elevated lead levels. Ira F. Brilliant Center for
Beethoven Studies, San José State University, CA.

It is clear that Beethoven's physicians were seriously limited in their available therapies, and that some of the treatment he received was less than beneficial. However, his doctors were using the best treatments available. Moreover, Beethoven, as even Schindler makes clear, was not the easiest of patients. He was critical, demanding, and at times even condescending toward his physicians. He often disagreed with their recommendations and was not compliant with their treatments. This in turn frequently led to a rupture in his relationship with the current physician. Managing a patient with Beethoven's kaleidoscope of medical problems would be a major challenge even for a twenty-first-century physician who had available a full range of modern technological, pharmacological, and psychosocial treatment facilities.

CHAPTER FOUR

The Interpretation

Such experiences (of not being able to hear) almost made me despair, and I was on the point of putting an end to my life – The only thing that held me back was my art. For indeed it seemed impossible to leave this world before I had produced all the works that I felt the urge to compose.

From the Heiligenstadt Testament, October 1802[1]

BACKGROUND

The earliest portions of the extensive literature in German, English, and French on Beethoven's medical problems dates from shortly after his death; there was a particular burst of publications around the centenary of his death in 1927, and it continues to grow. Much of the writing about Beethoven's health by both physicians and non-physicians is focused on his deafness, due to the dramatic poignancy of a composer who is unable to hear the sound of his own music. Many writers have also attempted to understand his other medical disorders, particularly his emotional problems and the cause(s) of his death, and there has been much speculation, if little consistency, in the medical interpretation of the diseases from which Beethoven suffered.

Researchers face a number of difficulties in attempting to place Beethoven's problems in a modern medical context. The absence of hard scientific data, such as biochemical or histological results, means that we are dependent on the more limited information provided in the surviving primary sources: the complaints he himself reported and the observations and records that others made about his health. This lack of detail has undoubtedly contributed to speculation about his medical disorders. There has been a tendency to isolate one symptom (such as deafness or diarrhea) or one autopsy finding (such as changes in the liver, pancreas, or kidneys) and build a diagnostic edifice on that finding, ignoring the existence of other clinical features that may not fit that interpretation. There has been a tendency also to rely on secondary rather than primary sources, particularly in discussions as to whether or not Beethoven had syphilis.

In this chapter I will examine each of the medical systems that were affected by his illnesses and will propose the most probable diagnosis, along with other possibilities, based on the clinical and autopsy evidence presented in chapter 3. The diagnoses proposed in both the medical and the non-medical literature will be outlined, with emphasis given to physician reports. Some diagnoses can be made with more conviction than others, and an attempt will be made to convey these differing shades of certainty.

THE AUTOPSY AND BEETHOVEN'S TERMINAL ILLNESS

The most striking changes at autopsy were found in the abdomen. There was a large amount of fluid in the peritoneal cavity (which of course was known before his death), and the liver, spleen, kidneys, and possibly the pancreas showed abnormalities visible to the naked eye.

The reduction in the size of the liver, its colour, "leathery" consistency, and the "bean-sized" nodules that covered its surface are all features typical of Laënnec's cirrhosis (named for the physician who first described it). In Laënnec's cirrhosis the nodules are typically less than 1 cm in diameter (termed "micronodules"): "bean-sized" fits with this dimension. Cirrhosis is characterized by the accumulation of fibrous tissue around the microscopic cellular structures of the liver. The fibrous tissue in turn obstructs the veins, venules, and exocrine ducts through which the digestive and other substances produced by the liver pass on their way to the bile duct and into the duodenum and small intestine. The obstruction of the veins and the resulting rise in backward pressure is the chief cause of the accumulation of fluid in the anatomical areas drained by those veins – in this instance the lower limbs and the abdominal cavity. Dilated venules at the lower end of the esophagus – called esophageal varices – can rupture easily, causing bleeding; this may have been the cause of the bleeding that Beethoven experienced in May 1825 and on several occasions during his final illness. This increased pressure in the veins was likely also the cause of the enlarged spleen that was found at the autopsy. Jaundice is caused partly by the metabolic malfunction of the liver and partly by the blockage of the bile duct. Toxins normally removed from the blood stream by a healthy liver, therefore, accumulate in the blood and the body, giving the skin and eyes a yellow hue typically seen with jaundice. The majority of medical authors who have described and interpreted Beethoven's medical problems in the last thirty years – W. Ober, Edward Larkin, Hans Bankl and Hans Jesserer, A. Kubba and M. Young, Jean-Louis Michaux, Peter Davies, and M. Keynes – have agreed that the composer had cirrhosis of the liver.[2]

While there are four main causes of cirrhosis of the liver – cardiac, biliary, post-viral, and alcoholic – as well as a rare "miscellaneous" group of causes, including hemachromatosis and Wilson's Disease,[3] the ultimate, naked-eye appearance of the liver is similar in each case.

1   Cardiac: There is no evidence that the cause of Beethoven's cirrhosis was secondary to cardiac disease. There is no clinical evidence of cardiac disease and the condition of his heart at autopsy was reported as normal.

2   Biliary: This condition is secondary to the presence of gallstones in the bile duct that cause chronic obstruction of the outflow of bile from the bile duct. "Biliary gravel" was found at Beethoven's autopsy, but this is unlikely to have been the cause of his cirrhosis because the two episodes of jaundice (the first in 1821, and the

second during the four months leading up to his death) were relatively painless and were not accompanied by the symptoms of gallstone colic, including recurrent pain in the upper right quadrant of the abdomen; biliary colic was diagnosable in the state of medical knowledge in the early nineteenth century. In addition, the "biliary gravel" stones generally are not large enough to block the bile duct. Moreover, with biliary obstruction the body and organs at autopsy would have been stained a deep green by biliverdin, a toxin produced by the malfunctioning liver. Biliary obstruction is relatively rare cause of cirrhosis.

3   Post-viral: There is a possibility that Beethoven's condition was caused by post-viral hepatitis. The six-week episode of jaundice that occurred in 1821 may have been caused by a virus. This episode cleared completely, leaving the liver damaged but still functioning. The argument against a viral cause for Beethoven's cirrhosis is the fact that hepatitis B and C – the types that can become chronic and cause cirrhosis – are late twentieth-century diseases, whereas hepatitis A – the type that almost never results in cirrhosis – prevailed in the nineteenth century. Hepatitis is usually accompanied by non-colicky pain in the abdomen, which Beethoven did not reportedly experience while he was jaundiced. Since hepatitis is diagnosed by carrying out biochemical tests and biopsy studies, it is not possible to prove or to disprove, at this juncture, that Beethoven's cirrhosis was post-viral. Three of the authors named above – Ober, Larkin, and Keynes[4] – favour post-viral hepatitis as the cause of his cirrhosis.

4   Alcohol: The final possibility is that the cirrhosis was induced by alcohol, which, until recently, was the cause of cirrhosis in approximately seventy-five percent of cases.[5] Both the amount of alcohol consumed and the length of time that the person has been drinking alcohol are key factors; a larger amount over a longer period is more likely to result in cirrhosis. However, personal factors, including genetic, immune, and liver physiology, also determine whether a particular individual consuming a

given amount of alcohol will develop cirrhosis. Malnutrition, including protein and vitamin deficiency, is another key factor that influences susceptibility. Cirrhosis, once it develops, is progressive if the person does not stop drinking. A number of physician-authors, including Kubba and Young, O'Shea, and P. Davies,[6] have concluded that the findings are consistent with alcoholic cirrhosis and this is the most favoured probable cause.

It is also possible that the cirrhosis was caused by a combination of infectious hepatitis and alcohol, a conclusion favoured by Bankl and Jesserer,[7] who argue that the episode of jaundice in 1821 has the typical features of infectious hepatitis because of its duration (six weeks) and because it was followed by diarrhea. Furthermore, the presence of hepatitis renders the liver sensitive to alcohol, so that smaller quantities will cause liver damage. However, liver disease due to alcohol can also cause transient jaundice followed by diarrhea. A present-day physician would require the finding of abnormalities on biochemical, immunological, and histological examination to confirm a diagnosis of infectious hepatitis. The possibility that Beethoven had this condition, therefore, cannot be either proved or disproved. The fact that hepatitis A, the type prevalent in the nineteenth century, rarely leads to cirrhosis makes this an unlikely cause of Beethoven's liver disease. The fact that the fluid in the abdominal cavity was "cloudy" and "reddish" suggests also that Beethoven may have had a spontaneous bacterial peritonitis associated with some bleeding. An inflammation of the membrane that lines the inside of the abdomen, peritonitis is a common complication of end-stage liver failure, and in the pre-antibiotic era, it would have been invariably fatal.

BEETHOVEN'S DRINKING HABITS

While the possibility that Beethoven may have overused alcohol has been proposed by some biographers and a number of physicians, including four of those who treated him, a definite conclusion has been met by the strongly worded arguments and opinions of some of the composer's friends and contemporaries, particularly Schindler, Wegeler, Ries, and Gerhard von Breuning, all of whom assert that Beethoven did not have an alcohol problem. Their opinions, however, are less persuasive when we examine their statements more closely.

Schindler's biography, published in 1840, thirteen years after Beethoven's death, is an invaluable source of material about Beethoven's life, but Schindler's style is hagiographic. For example, he refers to Beethoven as "our young hero"[8] or "our master,"[9] and he seems to have great difficulty in explaining Beethoven's eccentricities. He blames Beethoven's endless conflict with servants entirely on the servants,[10] and describes the "Immortal Beloved" letters in an elliptical manner, suggesting that this was a difficult issue for him as a biographer.[11] Schindler was reluctant to concede that Beethoven had any faults or flaws in his character or behaviour, and even carried this to the extent of distorting the truth or destroying evidence (such as correspondence and sections of the Conversation Books) that did not support his conclusions. For example, he states that he had shared accommodation with Beethoven when in fact he did not,[12] and he fabricated evidence to vilify Beethoven's nephew Karl, whom he disliked intensely.[13] Schindler was well aware that some of Beethoven's contemporaries, including Dr Wawruch and Karl Holz, believed that Beethoven drank to excess, and he attacked them vigorously from the outset; for example, Schindler alleges, falsely, that Wawruch called Beethoven a "drunkard brought by liquor to his final illness."[14] When discussing Beethoven's daily activities and diet, Schindler states that Beethoven's favourite beverage was spring water, which he drank in large quantities,[15] and adds that Beethoven liked wines from Budapest, particularly "the flavour of fortified wines which were very bad for his weakened stomach ... this fact alone is proof that Beethoven was not the drunkard his last doctor [Wawruch] claimed he was ... he often enjoyed a good glass of beer in the evening accompanied by his pipe and the paper ... [Wawruch] made defamatory remarks which gloss over his poor treatment."[16] Elsewhere, Schindler states: "It is very disconcerting to be asked if it was true that Beethoven found his inspiration in strong liquors ... even before the appearance of Wawruch's article this damaging rumour had been spread."[17] The Conversation Books include at least one entry where Schindler wrote to Beethoven, "You should not drink today," suggesting that even he may have been concerned at times by Beethoven's alcohol intake.[18] He conceded that Beethoven did drink to excess during the nine-month period from autumn 1825 until the summer of 1826, under the influence of Karl Holz, who had replaced Schindler as Beethoven's amanuensis for this period.[19]

These extracts from Schindler's biography and from the Conversation Books indicate that Schindler acknowledged that Beethoven enjoyed wine (including fortified wines) and beer, even if he was not a "drunkard" in the sense that he accuses Dr Wawruch of alleging. MacArdle (who translated and annotated Schindler's biography) concluded that Wawruch's opinions on Beethoven's indulgence in wine were "completely factual."[20] MacArdle notes that there is no evidence that Wawruch had accused Beethoven of being a "drunkard" as alleged by Schindler.

Wegeler's biography of Beethoven, written with Beethoven's pupil Ferdinand Ries and published in 1838, also criticizes Wawruch: "By and large, Beethoven lived moderately, and as far as I know, not one of his friends ever saw him intoxicated. Dr Wawruch's statement that Dr Malfatti had prescribed iced punch for him when he suffered from dropsy because, as an old friend, he knew of Beethoven's strong taste for alcoholic beverage, is therefore completely unfounded ... The accusation – which Livius had long ago leveled against musicians in Rome when he called them "vini avidum ferme genus" [people strongly taken to wine] and with which I frequently teased my friend – should be treated with considerable reservation."[21] However, since Wegeler saw little of Beethoven after the composer left Bonn for Vienna, he would not have had much personal knowledge of Beethoven's daily activities, behaviour, and lifestyle during the latter part of his life.

Gerhard von Breuning is critical of Dr Malfatti and Dr Wawruch, both for what he regarded as their poor medical care of Beethoven in his final illness, and because he disagreed with their opinion that Beethoven had a strong inclination for alcohol.[22] It will be recalled that Breuning, at age thirteen, was a frequent visitor to Beethoven in his final illness, and that his cheery and engaging exchanges, as recorded in the Conversation Books, brought a ray of light and hope to the composer's final, dreary months of life. Breuning subsequently became a well-known Viennese physician; he wrote and published his memoirs of Beethoven at the age of sixty in 1874. Breuning criticizes Wawruch and Malfatti's treatment of Beethoven's illness because they did not address the "root cause," but he does not explain what he believed the root cause to be or what he himself would have done in their situation. With the limited knowledge of the pathophysiology of liver failure available to them in 1827, Malfatti and Wawruch could not have done better than provide palliative terminal care, which they did to the best of their ability. Liver failure is a difficult condition to treat even with the full range of modern medical and surgical therapies.

Edward Larkin relies on the reports written by Schindler and Wegeler in drawing his conclusion that Beethoven did not have an alcohol problem.[23] Larkin notes that Wawruch's report was written after Beethoven's death, that Beethoven "loathed" Wawruch, and that Wawruch's report has all the marks of a "*causerie* on a favourite topic," and an "occasional piece" directed at a lay audience. Wawruch's complete report is given in Appendix 4, so readers can decide for themselves whether these criticisms are valid. However, as we have seen above, we have every reason to doubt Schindler's credibility on this issue, and Wegeler had little to do with Beethoven after the composer left Bonn. Wawruch's opinion on Beethoven's drinking habits, moreover, was shared by the three other physicians who treated him during the final seventeen years of his life: Malfatti, Braunhoffer, and Staudenheim.

W. Ober, another physician-author, also considered the possibility that Beethoven had an alcohol problem,[24] but concludes: "Neither his work habits, nor his conduct, supported the idea of alcoholism." In fact, some of Beethoven's behaviour *was* consistent with alcoholism: examples include his irritability, his poor self-care, and his lack of social graces, particularly in the later stages of his life. The possible effects of alcohol on his work habits and his creativity will be discussed in chapter 5.

The evidence of Karl Holz is also relevant. Holz was a competent amateur violinist who befriended Beethoven from August 1825 until December 1826, supplanting Schindler as Beethoven's unpaid secretary during this period. He was an outgoing and gregarious man who was able to help Beethoven socialize, and he was more candid and audacious in his relationship with Beethoven than was Schindler. In a letter to Otto Jahn in 1825 Holz states: "[Beethoven] was a stout eater of substantial food; he drank a great deal of wine at table, but could stand a great deal, and in merry company he sometimes became tipsy [*bekneipte er sich*]." In the evening he drank beer or wine (usually Voslau or red Hungarian wine). "When he had drunk he never composed. After the meal he took a walk."[25] Furthermore, Holz was not the cause of Beethoven's drinking, as alleged by Schindler, since Beethoven enjoyed taking substantial quantities of wine at times other than the period when he was associated with Holz.

That Beethoven's misuse of alcohol may have started as early as 1804 is suggested in a letter to Ferdinand Ries in July of that year in which Beethoven writes: "It is hard to forgive my worthy brother for not ordering the wine sooner since it is so necessary and beneficial to my health."[26] Although this statement is not an indication that Beethoven was overusing alcohol at that early stage, it does imply that he had a psychological need for it. In 1807 Dr Johann Schmidt, his physician at the time, counsels him to "drink moderate amounts of alcoholic beverages,"[27] and in 1811 Beethoven writes to Bettina Brentano, "I did not get home until four o'clock this morning from a bacchanalia, where I really had to laugh a great deal, with the result that today I have had to cry as heartily."[28]

Thayer provides two examples of Beethoven's misuse of alcohol in 1825.[29] The first occurred during a champagne party arranged to celebrate the visit of the Danish composer Friedrich Kuhlau to Vienna. In a letter to Kuhlau the next day, Beethoven wrote, "I must admit that the champagne went too much to my head also, yesterday, and again I was compelled to experience that such things retard rather than promote my capacities. For easy as it usually is for me to meet a challenge of the instant, I do not at all remember what I wrote yesterday." Thayer adds, without comment, that several pages of the Conversation Books recounting this event have been removed – torn out, perhaps, by a perspicacious Schindler? The second incident Thayer reports occurred in 1825 during a visit to Vienna of Sir George Smart, a well-known London musician and an admirer of Beethoven. Smart mentions Beethoven frequently in his memoirs and describes the dinner they had together. Earlier in the day, he notes, "I overheard Beethoven say, 'We will try how much the Englishman can drink.' *He* had the worst of the trial."[30] Smart gives no further details so it is unclear what having "the worst of the trial" means, but he does imply that Beethoven issued a challenge, at least to himself, to see whether Smart could drink more than he could.

The Conversation Books also provide information about Beethoven's enjoyment of and tolerance for wine. Many of the interactions took place in local taverns where Beethoven went for meals with his friends, and there are frequent comments and references to the wines at table. For example, in January 1820 an unknown person invites Beethoven to dinner and adds, "There will be eleven different types of wines."[31] Later in the same month Janitschek, while discussing a dinner party for the next day, states, "My wife is already cooking the oysters and adulterating ["*falsifier*"] the champagne ... the Bordeaux is much stronger than the Aldersburg." There are ten further references to wine during this month alone. On 21 March 1820 Bernard (a friend) tells Beethoven, "You drink too much wine."[32]

When evaluating whether or not a particular individual has an alcohol problem, a contemporary physician might ask the following questions: Do you drink in the mornings? Has the use of alcohol led to social or legal problems? Have others ever told you that you drink more than is good for you, or told you to stop? Are you able to stop taking alcohol?[33] We do not know whether Beethoven drank in the mornings. We do know that he was arrested on at least one occasion as a vagrant, although there is no indication that alcohol was involved. We know as well, from the above quotations, that at least some of his friends and four of his doctors believed that he drank more alcohol than was good for him, and that they advised him strongly to stop. We know also that he was not able to do so. The conclusion that Beethoven drank sufficient wine to affect his health is supported by Peter Davies in his scholarly work.[34]

The Diagnostic and Statistical Manual System of classifying psychiatric disorders (DSM-IV) recognizes two categories of alcohol disorder:

"dependence" and "abuse" (see Appendix 3). Dependence is characterized by increased tolerance for alcohol, withdrawal symptoms when the
alcohol is stopped suddenly, and use of "larger" amounts over a "longer"
period. There may also be unsuccessful efforts to cut down the intake, and
effects on lifestyle and health. "Abuse" is characterized by "major" effects
on social roles, and recurrent legal and/or interpersonal problems resulting from its use. Individuals with either of these conditions often have
predisposing genetic and personality traits, such as depressive, dependent, or hostile tendencies. It is likely that Beethoven had at least three
(the required minimum) of the seven criteria of "dependence": increased
tolerance, use of larger amounts over a longer period, and unsuccessful
efforts to cut down the intake, but he did not meet the criteria for alcohol
"abuse." Beethoven had both familial and psychosocial predisposing factors that could have contributed to a tendency to overuse alcohol. Both
his father and his paternal grandmother died of alcohol-related problems
– and we now know that there is a substantial genetic and familial component to alcoholism. There is also a statistical correlation between alcohol
misuse and single status, male sex, and psychological maladjustment: all
these predisposing factors were present in Beethoven's case.

Additional evidence comes from the results of the recent toxicological analysis of Beethoven's hair.[35] Russell Martin speculates that the high
levels of lead identified in the hair sample could have resulted from drinking mineral water at spas, from dishes, or from wine stored in lead-lined
flasks or lead crystal. He also considers "plumbed" wine (to which lead
was added to prevent bitterness) as a possible source. A final speculation
is that the lead in the hair sample was an artifact – that is, it was caused by
post-mortem contamination; assays of lead levels in post-mortem samples
of hair may not reflect plumbism because of ante-mortem or post-mortem
contamination.[36]

PLUMBED WINE

Documentation in French medical texts of the early nineteenth century
indicate that in that period of history wine merchants added lead salts

to wine in order to freshen or sweeten them and to delay or reverse their going sour.[37] The French physician François Merat notes that drinking wine adulterated with lead could cause "metallic colic," and that this action was fraudulent because it was illegal to add lead to wine.[38] Merat found that wine salesmen who added lead to wine were often the first victims of their "evil blending" (*perfides mélanges*),[39] and he notes that wine drinkers were also susceptible.[40] According to Merat the symptoms of "metallic colic" were colicky abdominal pains, nausea, and vomiting in the absence of fever. In severe cases there might be muscle weakness or even paralysis, particularly in the upper limbs, but this, he notes, was not common. About ten percent of patients who had metallic colic died from the condition (five of the fifty-seven cases in his series). In other cases, the disease followed a fluctuating course that could last for years. Merat also refers to an English author, Wilson, who described poisoning resulting from the inhalation of dust contaminated with lead in mines.[41] Merat describes six experiments carried out on wine that had been adulterated with "*litharge*" (lead oxide): the first was a practical taste test of wine to which a quantity of lead had been deliberately added; the remaining five experiments were chemical tests of wine, urine, and stool to determine whether lead was present. Because there is some repetition of method in the six experiments, only the first, second, and fourth are paraphrased below (my translation).

Experiment 1: A bad red wine was chosen ("the worst that could be found because these are the ones that are adulterated"). It had a pungent odour, and its flavour was sour and acrid. Twelve grains of litharge (lead oxide) were allowed to dissolve in this bottle of wine over a forty-eight-hour period. By then it had lost its austere, bitter flavour and had developed a sweet and pleasant taste. Two bottles of this wine would contain twenty-four grains of litharge, which is sufficient to cause metallic colic.

Experiment 2: When sulphuric acid was added to non-adulterated wine, it produced only a slight colour change. If it was added to leaded wine, a white precipitate formed, which settled in the bottom of the glass.

Experiment 4: When hydrogen sulphide ("*hydrogène sulphuré*") was added to leaded wine, a dark, flocculent deposit was produced. This was a sensitive test that could be used for medico-legal purposes when there was only a small quantity of lead in the wine.

In a two-volume monograph published only three years later and directed primarily to the lay public, Étienne Tourtelle[42] describes the harmful effects of drinking wine to which lead oxide has been added. He states: "It is very dangerous, it is a real poison and can shorten life ... its effects are pernicious." Tourtelle describes another method of identifying the presence of lead in wine, which was to allow the fluid to evaporate so that the remaining lead residue could be easily identified. He also comments that drinking excessive quantities of leaded wine could irritate the nervous system and affect the abdominal organs, causing dropsy and liver failure; the viscera could become "dried out," as was proved by "opening the bodies of those who worship Bacchus."[43] Recent books on the history of wine and wine making confirm that during this period lead was illegally added to wine to sweeten it and to prevent it from souring. Hugh Johnson[44] describes this as a "tragic legacy from ancient Rome" and refers to Eberhard Göckel, a "methodical and perspicacious" doctor from Ulm, Germany, who described its poisonous effects by tasting a sample of wine to which lead had been added and noting that subsequently he developed abdominal colic. The Duke of Wurtemburg subsequently passed an edict, with severe penalties attached, in which he condemned the use of lead in wine, but this information was suppressed by wine merchants. During the eighteenth century most countries passed laws prohibiting the use of lead salts in wine manufacturing, but this did not prevent its continued widespread use: for example, in 1750 Paris police discovered that a large quantity of spoilt wine brought to the city had been sweetened with lead oxide and sold.[45]

It is clear from these texts that wine to which lead salts had been added as a sweetener and a preservative was a cause of lead poisoning at least until the early nineteenth century. We do not know, and cannot prove, that the wine that Beethoven drank had been adulterated with lead salts.

It is probable that this was done only to cheap wines, and although we do have some indication of the types of wine that he enjoyed, we cannot conclude that they were contaminated. It is reasonable, however, to infer that such wine would be the most likely source of the lead found in his hair.

The clinical effects of lead poisoning caused by inorganic lead salts are colicky abdominal pains, constipation, and anemia; in more severe cases it affects the nervous system, causing nerve paralysis and mental confusion.[46] The most common nerve paralysis affects the radial nerve in the forearm, resulting in "wrist drop" – an inability to extend (straighten) the wrist joint; in rare cases it can affect other nerves, including the auditory nerve. Lead taken into the body is metabolized by various tissues, including the bones; lead can be identified in the bones of individuals exposed to lead poisoning long after they have ceased absorbing lead. A toxicological analysis of Beethoven's skeletal remains would help to clarify whether the lead found in his hair was an artifact or the result of ingestion of lead salts or products.

It should be noted that Beethoven did not display all the signs of alcohol dependency. None of his physicians mention that he had a tremor – a common feature of alcoholism – although this does not mean that no tremor was present. Furthermore, chronic alcohol abuse commonly affects the nervous system, but Beethoven retained his cognitive (intellectual) faculties until the last few days of his life. Indeed, he composed some of his most inspired music during his final years. It is therefore likely that his central nervous system was left relatively unimpaired by the toxic effects of alcohol.

Another feature requiring explanation is that Beethoven had a six-week episode of jaundice in 1821, five and a half years before his death. Jaundice can occur in either post-hepatitic or alcoholic cirrhosis. It is possible that his illness was caused by alcohol-induced hepatitis, a common precursor of cirrhosis, and that full-blown cirrhosis only developed later. The liver has substantial powers of regeneration. If enough functioning liver tissue is left, and the toxin is reduced or removed, it is possible for the liver to regain at least some of its function. Dr Staudenheim, Beethoven's physician at the time, insisted on strict obedience to his orders. We know from

Beethoven himself that after his jaundice had subsided he was treated with medicines and sent away to take the waters at Baden.[47] We know also that Dr Staudenheim advised Beethoven to stop drinking alcohol at this time: during a visit from Dr Braunhofer, who is at that point banning wine from the composer's diet, Karl writes in the Conversation Books, "Dr Staudenheimer [sic] also banned all wines."[48] This recommendation is also consistent with what was known about jaundice and liver pathology at the time. It is reasonable to infer that on the advice of Staudenheim, Beethoven did reduce his alcohol intake, at least for a time after the attack of jaundice in 1821, and that this allowed some liver regeneration to occur, extending his life expectancy by a few years.

It must be emphasized that a conclusion that Beethoven likely died of alcohol-induced cirrhosis is not a moral judgment on the composer or his behaviour. It is clear that he was not a "drunkard" – otherwise there would not be debate as to whether he had an alcohol problem. It is possible for a susceptible individual to drink alcoholic beverages in sufficient amounts to cause liver damage without taking so much as to cause serious behavioural or neurological effects. Beethoven was an unhappy man who fought his demons of depression, anger, and frustration on many occasions during his lifetime. It is only a short step from these emotions to the point where an individual first seeks and then needs an active and readily available pharmacological substance that will help to alleviate such unpleasant feelings at least on a temporary basis.

KIDNEY DISEASE

The other striking abnormality found at autopsy was in the kidneys: "calcareous concretions" were found in each of the calices of the kidneys. Davies describes these findings as "pathognomonic" (that is, typical) of a condition known as renal papillary necrosis,[49] but some medical scholars disagree with this interpretation.[50] Papillary necrosis is a rare inflammatory condition of the kidneys found in people with diabetes mellitus, chronic alcoholism, and other conditions such as pyelonephritis and analgesic abuse.[51] Davies considers that for Beethoven this condition was provoked by acute onset diabetes brought on, in turn, by destruction of the insulin-producing cells as a result of acute pancreatitis. Beethoven did have some of the symptoms of diabetes – thirst, weight loss, and dehydration – but Davies states that the diabetes was not diagnosed because the only test for sugar in the urine (the cardinal sign of diabetes) at that time was to taste the urine, which was not done for obvious reasons. Studies show that diabetes is present in twenty-five percent of patients with renal papillary necrosis; hence seventy-five percent of cases occur in the absence of diabetes.[52] Against the hypothesis that Beethoven had papillary necrosis is the fact that it occurs in chronic rather than acute onset diabetes. We may therefore conclude that although Beethoven likely did have renal papillary necrosis, this condition was terminal and could have been due to chronic alcoholism in association with liver disease, even in the absence of pancreatitis and diabetes. Pancreatitis causes severe, recurrent abdominal pain. Although Beethoven did have abdominal pain in the early and terminal stages of his final illness, we know it was not severe enough to warrant the use of opiates, which were widely used at that time for the control of pain, because these substances were not found in the chemical analysis of his hair.[53] This makes the diagnosis of pancreatitis, and therefore diabetes, less likely.

GASTROINTESTINAL PROBLEMS

According to his letters, Beethoven began experiencing gastrointestinal (GI) symptoms even before he left Bonn in 1792; in a letter to Franz Wegeler he states, "The [hearing] trouble is supposed to have been caused by the condition of my abdomen which, as you know, was wretched even before I left Bonn, but has become much worse in Vienna where I have been constantly afflicted with diarrhea and have been suffering in consequence from an extraordinary debility."[54] In an anecdote from 1795, Wegeler describes Beethoven as suffering "pretty severe colic which affected him frequently." At the time, Beethoven was preparing for a benefit recital for widows, and Wegeler was able to relieve him with "simple remedies."[55] Beethoven's bowel problems continued throughout his life, with recurrent colicky abdominal pain, diarrhea, and occasionally nausea and vomiting. He must also have experienced constipation at times: in a letter to Dr Braunhofer he requests "stronger medicine but it must not be constipating."[56] In his post-mortem report about Beethoven, Wawruch notes that Beethoven experienced alternating periods of constipation and diarrhea. With our knowledge of the state of medicine in the early nineteenth century, and with Beethoven's known proclivities for taking medicines, it is probable that he used purgatives regularly and in large quantities.[57] Hence the GI symptoms may have been due in part to the effects of these medications. but this does not explain the nature of the underlying symptoms that led him to use purgatives. There are four possibilities:

1 Irritable bowel syndrome (IBS) is a common "functional" disorder of the bowel characterized by recurrent episodes of diarrhea and/ or constipation and abdominal pain;[58] the symptoms are often chronic and may last for years. Wawruch describes it in analogous terms: "Beethoven noticed that his digestion began to suffer ... an alternate obstinate constipation and frequent diarrhea."[59] IBS is classified as functional because there is no clear pathology, and the condition is thought to be caused by an autonomic nervous system imbalance that is influenced by psychological and emotional factors. In addition, there is an expanding literature on the role of infection in inducing IBS. The nature, pattern, chronicity, and lack of lethality of Beethoven's symptoms, together with the absence of visible changes in the bowel at autopsy, make this the most likely underlying condition. This conclusion is supported by both Bankl and Jesserer and Peter Davies.[60]

2 Lead toxicity commonly causes constipation in addition to colicky pains in the abdomen, but this symptom may be modified by the use of purgatives. Although lead poisoning may have contributed to Beethoven's bowel problems in his later life, it is an unlikely cause in his twenties and thirties. An individual with chronic lead poisoning over a period of thirty years would also develop other visible complications, such as wrist drop due to paralysis of the radial nerve in the forearm.[61] Since Beethoven did not have muscle

paralysis, it is most likely that lead poisoning was a contributory cause of GI problems only toward the end of his life.

3   Inflammatory bowel disease has been proposed as a cause of Beethoven's bowel problems, a theory that could also explain his hearing loss, as it can on occasion affect the ear.[62] However, inflammatory bowel disease is potentially a severe and disabling condition, particularly before modern medication such as corticosteroids became available. Inflammatory bowel disease would likely have caused anaemia (from blood loss in the stool), nutritional deficiencies, and other complications such as bowel obstruction. Although Beethoven likely became anaemic during his final illness he did not suffer from the other complications; inflammatory bowel disease is therefore an unlikely cause of his bowel symptoms.

4   Parasitic infestation has not previously been proposed as a cause of Beethoven's bowel symptoms. Bowel parasites, which are found in association with poor hygiene and self-care, can cause the bowel symptoms we know Beethoven experienced, and could have been identified as a cause during the early nineteenth century. However, bowel parasites can also cause specific symptoms such as itchiness, and most parasite infestations are easily diagnosable because of their visible effects in the stool. Although it seems unlikely that Beethoven's physicians would have missed this diagnosis, it remains a possibility.

In conclusion, it appears most likely that Beethoven's bowel problems were initially the result of irritable bowel syndrome, and that this pattern was later affected both by misuse of purgatives and by emotional and psychological distress. Colic and constipation caused by lead toxicity may have been a further complicating factor in his later years.

DEAFNESS

Beethoven's deafness has been extensively discussed in both medical and non-medical literature. Maynard Solomon gives a detailed description

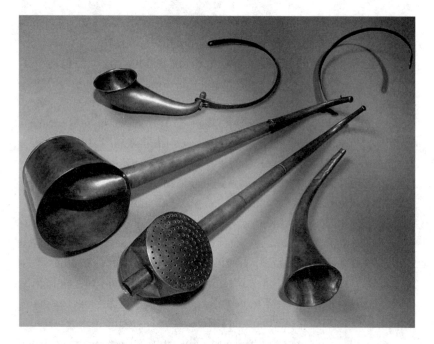

Beethoven's hearing aids. Beethoven-Haus, Bonn.

of the progress of Beethoven's deafness from the onset in 1798 and notes that as late as 1823 the composer retained some hearing capacity in his left ear and could hear loud speech and high tones.[63] Gerhard von Breuning observes that many people maintained that Beethoven was deaf only to speech and general noise but not to music.[64] However, Breuning relates an anecdote in which he entered Beethoven's room and began playing the piano; even though Breuning played quite loudly, Beethoven, who was deeply engaged in writing at his desk, showed no awareness of the sound. Breuning also notes that the Beethoven's Graf piano had an added amplification apparatus. From this, Breuning concludes that the composer was equally deaf to musical and non-musical sounds.

There is considerable evidence that Beethoven's deafness was not as complete as has been supposed, even toward the end of his life. A comprehensive review of his deafness and his use of ear trumpets and resonance plates has been described in the music literature. George Tomas Ealy notes that, with the aid of a sound conductor, Beethoven could hear himself playing at the keyboard until 1826; unfortunately the sound conductor has not survived so its effectiveness cannot now be tested.[65] Both Moscheles and Czerny reported that with the aid of an ear trumpet, Beethoven could hear some individuals' spoken speech until 1826. Ealy concludes: "Innovative adaptations characterize Beethoven's response to his hearing impediment. Using technology, he was able to hear throughout his adult life. The commonly held belief that he was functionally deaf can be dismissed." Despite these differing views of the extent of Beethoven's deafness, there is no disagreement that it had a major impact on his social life and musical career. What then are the possible causes of his deafness?

Acquired (as distinct from congenital) hearing loss may be conductive or sensorineural in nature. The cause of conductive hearing loss lies in the external or middle ear that "conducts" sound waves to the nerve receptors in the cochlea (the organ of hearing). The cause of sensorineural hearing loss lies in disease of the cochlea or the auditory nerve.[66] The two types can be distinguished by using a tuning fork to compare air and bone conduction: a person with conductive-type deafness can "hear" vibration when the tuning fork is placed on the mastoid bone, just below the ear, because the auditory nerve is still functional; a person with nerve deafness cannot hear this vibration.

Beethoven appears to have been sensitive to vibration. During the French army attack on Vienna in 1809 he hid in the basement with pillows covering his head and ears because he could not tolerate the cannon fire.[67] He seemed able to hear better when a device attached to the sounding board of his piano was connected to his temple to augment the vibrations.[68] His sensitivity to vibration suggests that the cause of his deafness was a middle-ear (conductive) rather than an auditory nerve condition. The most common cause of middle-ear deafness in middle-aged people is otosclerosis, a condition in which a thickening of the structures in the small bones of the middle ear impairs the responsiveness of the bones to sound. The fact that the onset of Beethoven's hearing loss was gradual, bilateral, and gradually progressive and that in the early stages it was accompanied by extra sounds (humming and buzzing) but not by pain is consistent with otosclerosis. Nothing was known about this condition in the early nineteenth century; the only treatment available was sound augmentation, which was provided as far as possible by the use of ear trumpets. Beethoven himself described the ear trumpet as very helpful in augmenting sound.[69]

Although otosclerosis is considered the most likely cause of his deafness, particularly in the German medical literature,[70] other researchers have proposed different conditions. Romain Rolland discussed Beethoven's symptomatology with Dr Marage, an ear, nose, and throat surgeon, who concluded that the cause was a combination of labyrinthitis and psychological factors due to Beethoven's ability to focus intensely on his music to the exclusion of other stimuli.[71] This condition would be equivalent to what we now call a conversion disorder, although Rolland does not use this phrase. Marage's interpretation also dovetails with Solomon's suggestion – based on Beethoven's own interpretation of the cause of his deafness – that the hearing loss may have been induced by his own rage.[72] However, this conclusion is unlikely because Beethoven's deafness in the last eight years of his life was dense and continuous; with conversion disorder it would have been variable and inconstant. M. Keynes has suggested that Beethoven's hearing loss was caused by Paget's Disease, which can cause deformity of the skull and involve the auditory nerve;[73] the autopsy did show a thickening of the bones of the skull, possibly caused by Paget's disease. However, this too is an unlikely cause since the hearing loss began at a much earlier age than is usual in this condition.

Various infectious and inflammatory causes for Beethoven's deafness have also been proposed. Davies has tabulated the many suggested diagnoses and concludes that there were multiple causes.[74] Beethoven is said to have had a "serious" illness, not mentioned in his correspondence, in 1797 or 1798, shortly before the onset of his hearing loss. Thayer notes that Dr Weisenbach, a surgeon from Salzburg who was also an acquaintance of Beethoven, considered that the composer had had an attack of typhus fever, which can occasionally cause deafness if it affects the auditory nerve.[75] The chronological relationship between the possible attack of typhus fever in 1797 and the onset of hearing loss in 1798 fits well with this theory. Another proposed cause is inflammatory bowel disease, since a sensorineural type of deafness is an occasional complication of this condition.[76] However, as noted above, it appears improbable that Beethoven had this condition since he showed none of the other generally severe effects of inflammatory bowel disease and because of the absence of blood in the stool. A further possibility is that the deafness was caused by lead poisoning: while it is unlikely that lead would have caused progressive hearing loss starting in his thirties without other accompanying neurological manifestations of toxicity, it may have been an exacerbating factor in his later life. The possibility that his deafness was caused by syphilis will be discussed below.

It is difficult to explain the changes found in Beethoven's auditory apparatus at autopsy. The significance of the increased vascularization of the cochlea is uncertain but may indicate an inflammatory process. The "wrinkled (auditory) nerves that lacked a central core" could be a sign that the nerves were atrophied: this can occur in otosclerosis where there is a loss of nerve cells located in the internal ear. Auditory nerve atrophy can result from a number of other conditions that cause deafness. Another finding in the autopsy report that has been little discussed in the medical literature was that the auricular arteries were "cartilaginous," by which the pathologist likely meant that walls of the arteries were hard, as occurs in atherosclerosis. This is not particularly relevant to his deafness, but if his auricular arteries were atherosclerotic, it is likely that arteries elsewhere were also affected, and at this degree of severity would be an unusual finding in a man of fifty-six. Although there are many causes of early-onset atherosclerosis, it commonly accompanies chronic liver disease secondary to alcoholism and would also have been aggravated by his smoking.

From this review of his deafness, the clinical presentation is most consistent with otosclerosis. However, if it could be established that Beethoven did, in fact, have typhus fever in 1797, auditory nerve disease resulting from this condition would remain a possibility.

PSYCHIATRIC AND PSYCHOSOMATIC SYMPTOMS

In his correspondence Beethoven complains most frequently of psychiatric and psychosomatic symptoms. His most common complaint is depression, but at other times he notes anxiety, insomnia, and anger. On two occasions he describes physical symptoms associated with, and likely the result of, anxiety (psychosomatic symptoms; see table 3.3). At times his depression was severe enough to bring on thoughts of death, and on two occasions – in 1810 and in 1817[77] – he mentions suicide or a wish to die by his own hand. He also mentions suicide in general terms in the Heiligenstadt Testament of 1802. It is not known whether he made any suicide attempts, but it appears unlikely. Most of his episodes of depression follow clear-cut events: for example, the death of his mother in 1787, the awareness of his hearing loss (1805 and 1810), the break-up of a relationship (1810), the death of his brother (1816), a conflict with servants (1817), and difficulties with his nephew Karl (1819, 1825, 1826), although on some occasions there does not seem to be a particular precipitating event (1809, 1813, 1817, 1822).[78]

When a psychiatrist makes a diagnosis, an attempt is made to distinguish between a condition considered a psychiatric illness and one associated with an individual's personality, a distinction reflected in the Diagnostic and Statistical Manual, fourth edition (DSM-IV), a system of classifying mental illness.[79] With the DSM-IV system a "diagnosis" is made on each of five axes: Axis I, a diagnosis of the primary psychiatric disorder; Axis II, a diagnosis of the personality disorder (if present); Axis III, a diagnosis of organic medical conditions; Axis IV, a report of psychosocial and environmental problems; and Axis V, a "global" assessment of functional level. In applying this diagnostic system to Beethoven, I will address Axis II followed by Axis I; Axis III diagnoses are discussed elsewhere in this chapter, and diagnoses on Axes IV and V will not be addressed.

There is little doubt that Beethoven had an eccentric personality. Many friends and acquaintances commented on and had difficulty with his character. He was extroverted, he spoke his mind with sometimes destructive candour, he was irascible, and he was critical even of his close friends.[80]

He was known on occasion to become involved in physical scraps with his brother Carl,[81] and on one occasion with a male servant.[82] However, once his anger had been vented, he would be remorseful and apologetic to an exaggerated extent.[83] As a result of these conflicts, he became estranged from even close friends, such as Stephan von Breuning or Anton Schindler, or his brothers, sometimes for years on end. Others who experienced his anger, such as Archduke Rudolf, had sufficient patience and respect for his genius to tolerate his tirades. His conflicts with servants were endless and repetitive, and friends, such as Countess Erdödy and Zmeskall, often had to intervene and help restore peace to the household. Similar conflicts with neighbours and landlords resulted in frequent, complex, and expensive changes of lodgings.

Beethoven was acutely sensitive to insult, resulting in a suspicious attitude bordering on the paranoid toward certain individuals or groups.[84] For example, he often referred to unspecified "enemies" in the Vienna musical scene; although there were undoubtedly some who disliked both him and his music, this enmity would seem exaggerated out of proportion to the situation. A paranoid attitude is not uncommon in individuals with an alcohol problem, and deafness can also increase paranoid attitudes and beliefs. Beethoven also had a maladroit attitude to money. Particularly toward the end of his life, he wrongly believed himself to be poor, and in letters often refers to his limited assets. Yet his frequent moves were costly and his legal bills, particularly between 1816 and 1820 when he was contesting custody of Karl, were very high. His negotiations with publishers – when he offered or even sold a composition simultaneously to two or more publishers – got him into expensive legal tangles.

Despite these difficulties, Beethoven had a good sense of humour. He enjoyed teasing his friends and in letters often made puns on the name of the person to whom he was writing. For example, Karl Holz was "Most excellent Chip" or "Most excellent piece of mahogany"[85] (Holz is the German word for wood). He was able to promote a remarkable degree of loyalty and devotion from friends such as Wegeler, Zmeskall, and Amenda, for whom he had lifelong affection. In spite of much rivalry and conflicts with both his brothers, he had an intense family feeling – Breuning calls it a "blind" love for his family – and his loyalty to Carl, and Carl's son Karl, lead him to questionable behaviour and tactics in his battle to obtain custody of Karl after his brother's death.

Do these characteristics add up to an Axis II diagnosis of a personality "disorder" in modern terms? DSM-IV defines personality disorders as having four characteristics:[86]

A   An enduring pattern of inner experience and behaviour that deviates markedly from the expectation of an individual's culture.

B   The enduring pattern is inflexible and pervasive across a broad range of personal and social situations.

C   The enduring pattern leads to clinically significant distress or impairment in functioning.

D   The pattern is stable and of long duration and can be traced back to adolescence or early adulthood.

In addition, the enduring pattern is not the result either of another mental disorder or of substance abuse. Beethoven likely meets criteria A, B and C but not D. With the exception of a tendency to irritability, there is little on record to suggest that his characterological problems started in adolescence or even in early adulthood. The first intimation we have of inappropriate behaviour and conflict with friends is the Heilegenstadt Testament of 1802 at age thirty-one. In addition, these behavioural changes seemed to become progressively worse as he aged, whereas the natural history of personality disorder is that it tends to improve with age, even without specific treatment. Thus, it would appear that Beethoven did not have a personality disorder per se, but rather that his progressive character difficulties were the psychological and social consequence of his increasing deafness and his misuse of alcohol as he grew older.

Did Beethoven have an Axis I diagnosis? The most likely Axis I diagnosis is that of Recurrent Depression. DSM-IV defines a major depressive episode as having the following characteristics over a two-week period:[87]

1   depressed mood most of the day nearly every day

2   diminished interest and pleasure

3   weight loss or weight gain

4   insomnia or hypersomnia nearly every day

5   agitation or retardation

6   fatigue

7   feelings of worthlessness and guilt

8   impaired concentration and decisiveness

9   thoughts of death

In addition, the symptoms must impair social functioning and are not caused by another medical or psychological event. Beethoven experienced hopelessness, suicidality, anxiety, somatic symptomatology, guilt, and insomnia. Although we cannot be certain whether his depressed episodes lasted two weeks or more, in the event that they did, the diagnostic criteria for major depression would be met.

It is more difficult to determine whether he had additional hypomanic episodes that would point to a diagnosis of Bipolar (or Manic-Depressive) disorder. DSM-IV defines a hypomanic episode as having the following characteristics:[88]

A   A period of elated, expansive or irritable mood lasting at least
     three days.

B   The elevated mood is accompanied by at least three of the
     following symptoms:

     1   inflated self-esteem or grandiosity

     2   decreased need for sleep

     3   increased talkativeness

     4   racing thoughts (expressed in words or writing)

     5   distractibility

     6   agitation

     7   increased pleasurable activities that may have painful
          consequences

In addition, the episode is accompanied by a change of functioning that is observable by others but is not severe enough to cause marked impairment of social functioning, and it is not the result of another medical or psychological condition. Beethoven's letters on occasion convey excitement and even euphoria; the following letter, addressed to Sigmund Steiner, one of his publishers, might be seen as an example of "racing thoughts" expressed in writing (the emphases are Beethoven's):

Most excellent General, The following letters are for <u>Schlemmer</u> and Haring. <u>The latter lives quite close to you in the Kohlmarkt, at the Schwabisches Haus</u>. Please deliver them at once, in the greatest haste, prestissimo, as speedily as possible; and sell those <u>sows</u> immediately. Volti subito

You are to hand over to the Adjutant everything pertaining to the violoncello I should like to have it clearly entered in the trio – Please report to me as soon as the trio is ready, so that I may send the Archduke a copy of it – you must hurry, therefore, presto, prestissimo; and spur on the Adjutant – If anyone sends me a letter, please forward it here citissime. Everyone is making haste so that the public exchequers may be filled and the General Staff be suitably entertained! – Schlemmer lives in the Kohlmarkt at the little Brandauisches Haus. It is important too that this scoundrel should receive his communication immediately – Volti subito. I hear that the song about "Merkenstein" is to appear during the skating season, i.e. Veni, Vidi, Vici!!! The Adjutant is still under suspicion in connexion with the score of the quartet. Hence I recommend the most thorough investigation. <u>I have had a look at it here, and it cannot be corrected without the score</u> – With all my heart I embrace the L[ieutenant] G[eneral] and wish him the penis of a stallion. In haste, the G[eneralissim]o.[89]

An earlier letter, written to Zmeskall in 1802, also suggests racing thoughts:[90]

My dearest Baron, Barone, Baron! – Domanovitz,
Please sacrifice one friendship to another today and come to the Schwan – You will therefore greatly oblige, Your etc.
Count Bthvn.
Baron? – Baron – ron – aron – ron– etc. Hail and happiness, happiness and hail and hail and happiness, happiness, hail, hail, happiness etc.
Baron

Baron

Baron

Baron

Several other letters to friends around this period have a similar racing and expansive flavour.[91] When he received notice that Therese Malfatti had turned down his offer of marriage, he responded: "Your news has plunged me from the heights of the most sublime ecstasy down into the depths."[92] These examples strongly suggest that Beethoven may have had transient hypomanic episodes, in which case it is likely that he suffered from what now would be called manic-depressive or bipolar disorder. His racing style is very similar to examples of writing in individuals with hypomania reported in the psychiatric literature.[93] Based on a review of his behaviour, Davies also concludes that Beethoven likely had transient hypomanic episodes.[94] It is notable that Beethoven's moods followed a strong seasonal pattern. His general health as well as his mood tended to be worse in the winter and better in the summer, and he frequently comments on this himself. As table 3.6 exemplifies, in his correspondence there are no references to "feeling better" either in mood or in health during the winter months. This strongly suggests that his depression had a seasonal pattern, although it does not indicate, in itself, that he had what we would now call a seasonal affective disorder.

The remaining Axis I diagnosis, as is clear from the discussion above and in chapter 3, is substance dependence: an excess use of wine and related products. Depression and alcohol dependence commonly occur together in the same individual. In some cases, depression occurs first and is followed by a development of alcohol dependence; in others alcoholism sets the initial pattern and is followed by depression. Whatever the order, a vicious cycle is established where the individual self-medicates depressive symptoms with alcohol, which, because it is a nervous system depressant, in the end, aggravates the depression. Since references to depression first appear at an earlier stage in Beethoven's life than references to the misuse of alcohol, we can conclude that his alcoholism was likely secondary to an affective disorder, rather than a primary condition.

The coexistence of depression and alcoholism in the same individual is indicative of a more serious prognosis than either of the two conditions alone. Suicidality also is more prevalent in this situation.

RESPIRATORY PROBLEMS

Although Beethoven experienced regular "colds" (upper respiratory tract infections), his respiratory problems appeared to coalesce around two discrete occasions in his life: the first following his mother's death from tuberculosis in 1787, and the second following his brother Carl's death in November 1815, also from tuberculosis. After his mother's death, he developed what he called "asthma," although this condition cleared within a short time. Following his brother's death, he complained of a number of symptoms, beginning with "heavy colds" and a "feverish cold," followed later by a cough; his condition was eventually diagnosed in July 1817 as a "disease of the lungs," although the type and character of the disease were not specified either by Beethoven or in any other primary source. Dr Staudenheim, his physician at the time, was clearly perplexed by this illness. This led to Beethoven's statement that his doctor had "finally" diagnosed disease of the lungs,[95] but even this final diagnosis seems tentative: "disease of the lungs" could describe almost any lower respiratory condition. It appears that the illness was not accompanied by potentially serious respiratory symptoms, such as hemoptysis (coughing up blood) or dyspnea (shortness of breath). Beethoven first refers to a cough in December 1817, and thereafter mentions it with increasing frequency. Conditions such as bronchitis, tuberculosis, and pleurisy were diagnosable in the state of medical knowledge at the time but were not mentioned as possibilities.

Beethoven was a moderate pipe smoker and later in life he enjoyed cigars.[96] Between 1819 and 1826 he complained of catarrh and cough on five occasions. It is therefore probable that during these later years he developed bronchitis, caused or aggravated by pipe and cigar smoking, even though neither he nor any of his physicians used this diagnostic phrase. Davies also suggests this diagnosis.[97] It is possible that his initial pulmonary symptoms following his brother's death were caused by anxiety about his own health resulting from identification with the illness and death of his brother rather than from any clearly defined physical disease. This possibility appears reasonable because Beethoven had developed similar symptoms of asthma (or tightness of the chest) and "melancholia" following the his mother's death twenty-seven years previously. However, once the cough and "catarrh" (likely bronchial mucus) began in 1818–19, bronchitis induced by smoking becomes a more probable diagnosis. The fact that no naked-eye abnormalities of the lungs were identified at his autopsy eight years later is also consistent with these conditions.

EYE SYMPTOMS

The eye symptoms are perhaps the most difficult of Beethoven's medical problems to understand because he describes them in such non-specific terms, and because there is no other primary source for their appearance and character. Beethoven refers to eye symptoms in his letters on seventeen occasions over a nine-month period, between April 1823 and January 1824; during most of this period, he was completing his work on the ninth symphony. He states that his eyes are "sore," that he saw everything "only very slowly," and that these problems interfered with his writing. It was worse in town air, and it would clear quickly "if I did not wear glasses." Toward the end of this period, his condition was improving and he states that he can now use his eyes by daylight.

From these complaints we can infer that he experienced pain and photophobia but not lacrimation, discharge, or redness. The condition clearly affected both eyes and cleared completely; after January 1824 he never again refers to eye problems. The most probable diseases that would present with this constellation of symptoms in a middle-aged man are uveitis and scleritis, inflammatory conditions of the uveal tract and the sclera respectively.[98] Although there often are underlying causes for these conditions, including infection, auto-immune disease, or malignancies, they can also be "idiopathic," that is, they occur incidentally, with no apparent underlying cause. Interstitial keratitis, an inflammatory condition that

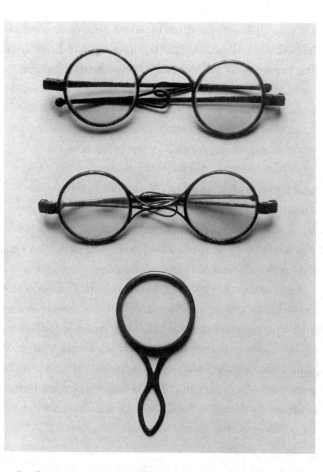

Beethoven's spectacles and eyeglass. Beethoven-Haus, Bonn.

affects the cornea, has been proposed as a possible cause of his eye problems,[99] but this condition is usually part of a systemic or infective process
such as tuberculosis, leprosy, syphilis, or some viral infections; there is
little evidence that Beethoven had any of these diseases. Another possible
cause is a seasonal allergy syndrome affecting the eye. In favour of this
possibility is the fact that the condition seems to have started in April and

had largely subsided by September. However, when this condition affects the eye it is usually accompanied by lacrimation, and Beethoven appears not to have experienced this symptom. Unless or until further evidence is forthcoming, idiopathic uveitis or idiopathic scleritis remain the most probable causes of Beethoven's eye problems.

MUSCULOSKELETAL SYMPTOMS

In 1821 and again in 1826 Beethoven refers to "rheumatism,"[100] and on two occasions his doctors state that he has gout.[101] During the early nineteenth century the word "rheumatism" was used as a general term to describe localized or generalized muscle and joint pain.[102] A diagnosis of rheumatism at that time would include conditions that we know as osteoarthritis, rheumatoid arthritis, and fibromyalgia. The early nineteenth-century description of gout, on the other hand, is similar to our current understanding of the condition, and the association of gout with a disturbance of uric acid metabolism was also known at that time.[103] From the little we know about Beethoven's symptoms and signs, it is unlikely that he had gout, but he may have had fibromyalgia, a condition that we now know is commonly associated with both depression and irritable bowel syndrome.

OTHER POSSIBLE MEDICAL PROBLEMS

In recent years physicians have put forward a number of other medical conditions that might have affected Beethoven,[104] including mercury poisoning,[105] sarcoidosis,[106] systemic lupus erythematosus,[107] and Whipple's Disease,[108] amongst others. Of these, the only one with some degree of probability is sarcoidosis, a condition that can affect many bodily systems including lungs, skin, joints, eyes, liver, and lymph nodes. However, since sarcoidosis does not cause death from liver failure and the appearance of the liver and lungs at the autopsy were not those of sarcoidosis, this possibility is unlikely.

None of these diseases are common, and their diagnosis is not easy, even with the availability of modern laboratory facilities. The reasoning behind such proposals is an attempt to explain all Beethoven's medical problems under one diagnostic category. While this is a commendable objective, in most instances the suggestions are speculative, and it is not possible to either prove or disprove them. Clarence Merskey, a distinguished clinical teacher and internist at the University of Cape Town, frequently repeated the following aphorism: "Common conditions occur commonly." This statement is self-evident, but is nevertheless often forgotten by medical diagnosticians intent on making obscure clinical diagnoses. A similar argument was also used in a debate as to whether Vincent van Gogh had manic-depressive illness or porphyria:[109] the former affects one percent of the population and the latter only 0.008 percent. Because manic-depression is so much more prevalent in the population, the authors argued strongly that Van Gogh likely suffered from this condition. Both depression and alcohol dependency are common conditions. The historical evidence in Beethoven's case suggests that he suffered from both conditions and that his use of alcohol in the form of wine and beer led to the liver disease from which he died.

THE SYPHILIS MYTH

Gossip about the possibility that Beethoven had syphilis started shortly after his death, but the belief that he had this condition only became widespread after the publication of the first edition of the influential *Dictionary of Music and Musicians*, edited by George Grove.[110] Grove wrote the entry on Beethoven, and in a footnote he states that Dr Lauder Brunton, a medical friend whom he consulted, had confirmed this belief and had stated that the post-mortem appearances were those of syphilis. Grove did not provide Brunton's credentials, but he was a well-known internist in his day. Grove also states that the diagnosis of syphilis was confirmed by the existence of two prescriptions for this disease reported to Thayer by Dr Bertolini. Grove does not identify the prescriptions or indicate what medication was being ordered. It will be recalled that Bertolini was Dr Malfatti's assistant and that he treated Beethoven between 1808 and 1816. Thayer interviewed Bertolini and in his biography on Beethoven recounts an anecdote from the doctor about Beethoven, but this anecdote does not include mention of a prescription or of syphilis.[111] Speculation on the diagnosis of syphilis reached a peak with the publication of Ernest Newman's book on Beethoven in 1927;[112] Newman not only believed that Beethoven had syphilis, but also alleges that Thayer deliberately concealed information he had received from Dr Bertolini about this diagnosis. It is also possible that Thayer heard allegations about Beethoven's syphilis but decided that they were not substantial enough to recount in his landmark biography.

Although syphilis can mimic many different medical conditions, it does not cause the clinical and pathological features of Beethoven's ill health, such as recurrent episodes of colic and diarrhea, transient respiratory symptoms, and cirrhosis of the liver. On occasion, syphilis can cause auditory nerve neuropathy resulting in deafness, and it can also affect the eye, but ear and eye infection do not occur as isolated phenomena unaccompanied by other signs of the disease. Syphilis can affect the skin, cause genito-urinary lesions (particularly if it is associated with gonorrhea as is often the case), produce visible tumours (gummas) in various parts of the body, and in its advanced stages cause serious cardiac and cerebral pathology. In rare cases it can affect the liver, producing visible and characteristic changes known as "hepar lobatum." These changes were not found at Beethoven's autopsy, and Wawruch makes no mention of syphilis in his report on Beethoven's medical history (see Appendix 4): if syphilis had been present, Wawruch would likely have known about it, and his frankness about Beethoven's misuse of alcohol indicates that he was not trying to put a gloss on Beethoven's medical problems. Finally, the fact that the hair analysis showed no evidence of the presence of mercury, which at that time was the treatment for syphilis, supports the conclusion that Beethoven did not have this disease. Recent reviews of the evidence that Beethoven suffered from syphilis made by physicians have concluded that the possibility is hypothetical at best.[113]

A well-written and provocative monograph by Deborah Hayden gives strong support to the possibility that Beethoven had syphilis.[114] Hayden describes the history of syphilis, its first appearance in Europe after 1492, and its rapid spread and prevalence thereafter, and provides case histories of famous individuals, including Beethoven, whom she believes may have had the disease. She considers that the multiplicity of his health problems and his "high risk" behaviour of consorting with prostitutes are consistent with this conclusion. However, the evidence that he consorted with prostitutes is circumstantial[115] and is not supported by all scholars.[116] Moreover, the mode of his death was chronic liver failure, not heart failure or brain disease, as would be the case with syphilis. The autopsy findings, limited as they were, did not reveal signs of syphilis such as brain atrophy, reddened and inflamed meninges, heart enlargement, aortic aneurysms, or gummas, all of which would have been visible to the naked eye had they been present. Thus, the clinical evidence that Beethoven had syphilis is minimal, and the autopsy evidence is absent. It is time for the myth that Beethoven had this condition to be permanently laid to rest.

CONCLUSIONS

Conclusions about the etiology and diagnosis of the medical problems suffered by Ludwig van Beethoven must, because of the nature of the situation, remain conjectural. The evidence that we have from his letters, his friends, and the limited nature of his physician's reports is incomplete and sometimes conflicting. Decisions need to be based, as in a court of law, on the balance of probabilities. Nevertheless, if the known facts are put together, it is possible to come to reasonable, evidence-based conclusions.

No single clinical syndrome, other than very rare conditions, can explain all of Beethoven's problems. It is more probable that he had a number of conditions, both psychiatric and medical. There is a strong possibility that he had recurrent depressive episodes, and it is also likely that he had what would now be called a bipolar disorder. Otosclerosis is the likely cause of his deafness, and he also suffered from irritable bowel syndrome. Late in life he may have had had lead poisoning, but the presence of high lead levels in his body is yet to be confirmed by a toxicological analysis of his skeletal remains. The cause of death was liver failure due to cirrhosis caused by a long-term misuse of alcohol in the wine and beer he consumed, complicated in the final stages by failure of kidney function. The conclusion that he died from alcohol-induced liver failure would remain even if it were shown that the high levels of lead found in his hair were artifactual – derived from external contamination – rather than from the use of plumbed wine.

Beethoven's prodigious energy enabled him to overcome problems that would have crushed a lesser mortal. His soaring spirit enabled him to compose music that expressed joy, peace, and spirituality even when his body was wracked with disease and when he was isolated and insulated from people and from sound. We can but marvel that his creative genius continued to be expressed, and that, until shortly before the onset of his terminal illness, he was able to plumb the depths of feeling in his music.

CHAPTER FIVE

Illness and Creativity

Plaudite, amici, comoedia finita est. (Applaud, friends, the comedy is finished.)
Beethoven's words on his deathbed.[1]

Art and culture are the distinguishing and most enduring marks of a civilization. We know little about Cro-Magnon man and other prehistoric peoples other than what they chose to depict on the walls of their caves or in their architecture and pottery. In more recent historic times the art, architecture, and writings of ancient Egyptian, Greek, Roman, early Chinese, Amerindian, African, and other civilizations provide a revealing glimpse of the interests, activities, and daily lives of these peoples. The same can be said of our civilization: our art will be remembered and admired by future generations when many other distinctive artifacts and structures are forgotten or destroyed. The National Aeronautics and Space Administration (NASA) recognized the symbolism of art in our present-day earthly civilization by including a recording of Glenn Gould playing Johann Sebastian Bach's *Goldberg Variations* among the artifacts sent into deep space on the *Voyager* mission in 1979.

Music is distinctive as an art form because, unlike literature or even painting, it has no clear connection with human communication. It evokes emotions and feelings and its appreciation and beauty depend more on this visceral quality than on its cognitive appeal. Singing, dancing, and the playing of musical instruments such as drum, flute, lyre, and didgeridoo were part of the traditional cultures of early civilizations, but a historical tradition requires the development of musical notation, which did not happen until the eleventh and twelfth centuries in western civilizations.[2] The use of a written musical language stimulated the development of instrumentation and added to the variety of musical forms and the originality and complexity of sound combinations.

The psychology of creativity and its relationship to psychiatric and medical illness is an area of great interest. What factors are related to creativity? How may it be promoted and what inhibits creativity? How can psychological and medical concepts be used to provide a better grasp of the principles and processes on which creativity is based? Information on these topics will shed light on our understanding of the relationship between Beethoven's health problems and his creativity and will help our attempt to answer the question, "How was it possible for Beethoven to compose a vast volume of awe-inspiring music while suffering so many serious, complicated, and chronic illnesses?"

In his excellent monograph on Beethoven's compositional process, Barry Cooper describes Beethoven's extensive use of "sketches" in the preparation of the final draft of a work.[3] Much of his composition was done out of doors, and he always carried a notebook so that he could write down musical ideas as soon as they occurred. He also had a tendency to sing or hum while composing. The sketchbooks served as an essential aide-memoir, and the singing and humming (and piano-playing while it was still audible to him) provided feedback on the sound of the written notes. The sketchbooks reveal that Beethoven strove for musical perfection: he wished to create something that was not only beautiful and artistic but also novel and surprising.[4]

THE PSYCHOLOGY OF CREATIVITY

The last fifty years has seen a rapid growth in both research and writing on creativity.[5] Creativity is a complex subject and, at least partly because of this complexity, it has generated much speculation. As with many other topics in the field of knowledge, the lack of information has not prevented – and may even have helped to provoke – a torrent of discussion about the nature, causes, and effects of creativity. It is useful to distinguish "every-day" creativity from "eminent" creativity.[6] Everyday creativity is common and may even be universal in the human species, whereas eminent creativity is rare and involves widespread social acceptance of the creative performance of an individual. Eminent creativity, which is our main concern here, is the type that is widely coupled with the concept of genius.

Creativity must have an end-product, whose originality and usefulness are its two defining features:[7] the created product must be novel and original; it must also be appropriate and have value or utility. Creative arts such as painting, music, or literature are obvious examples of creativity, and the value of the product is often described in terms of its beauty, appeal, and attractiveness. This leads to the vexing question of what constitutes "beauty" in the creative arts. Does beauty have distinctive and objective quality or, as cynics suggest, does it exist only in the eye of the beholder? The visual or auditory impact of an artwork on the "beholder" must be part of the definition of beauty; if the audience is sufficiently large, the artist might achieve "eminent" status. However, there also are objective criteria for beauty: for example, many would regard the reconciliation of opposites, such as occurs in the symmetry, originality, and complexity of the created object, as essential components of beauty.[8] Even the intangible domain of ideas may be the product of creativity. One of the most famous creative acts of the twentieth century is Einstein's formula on relativity: initially this was a purely theoretical concept, but it opened the doors to a wealth of information on the structure and dynamics of the universe and of molecular and atomic function.

Personal traits, such as devotion to work, independence, drive for originality, and flexibility are key requirements for creativity. Hayes[9] found that creative individuals showed a strong tendency towards independent action and had the capacity to mix different strategies in finding solutions to problems. He emphasized the importance of preparation time to eminent creativity. In a sample of 500 compositions written by seventy-six great composers, he found that only three of the works were written earlier than the tenth year of the composer's career; there was a similar although shorter preparation time among painters and poets. During this early period of preparation, the artists learn, work, and acquire the skills necessary for their art. Beethoven's career was launched with his first visit to Vienna in 1787, and his first noteworthy compositions were the early piano sonatas and piano trios completed in 1795. His "preparation time" was thus eight years, a slightly shorter period than that predicted in Hayes' hypothesis.

Hayes also emphasizes that the features that most clearly differentiate creative from non-creative people are motivational rather than cognitive. The vital importance of motivation and application in creativity was well expressed by Thomas Edison, who, in an interview with *Life Magazine* in 1932, stated that creativity was "ninety-nine percent perspiration and one percent inspiration." This pithy aphorism underlines the importance of hard work and seemingly downgrades the inspirational idea. However, this may be more apparent than real. Many artists, philosophers, and inventors have experienced the "Eureka!" phenomenon – the flash of insight and inspiration that occurs when a great truth is discovered, or a complex problem resolved.[10] Edison's maxim makes more sense if we consider the time involved. While the flash of insight takes seconds, the working time taken to get to that point may be measured in months or years. "Perspiration" may therefore be an essential prerequisite for "inspiration." Hard work likely arouses an unconscious, problem-solving process that causes the "Eureka!" phenomenon to occur as the solution hits the conscious mind. Creative artists are people with energy, goals, and vision. They have an urge that both impels and compels them to externalize ideas and concepts. The enthusiasm with which these efforts are pursued varies in different artists and in the same artist at different times, but the ability to apply oneself vigorously to a task with distant and uncertain goals is indispensable. For this reason, creative individuals are often demanding of themselves and of others.

Even dreams may stimulate creativity. During the course of art therapy, Almuth Lutkenhaus-Lackey, the well-known German-born Canadian sculptor, described how her dreams provided ideas for her artistic creations.[11] During her dreams she saw faces and symbols that reminded her of traumas of her early childhood in Germany during the Second World War. She was able to use these visions and the feelings they aroused as a starting point to recreate her experiences in drawing and sculpture. This, in turn, enabled her to "work through" her childhood traumas by creating works of great originality and beauty. Beethoven also describes inspiration that came in a dream:

While I was dozing I dreamt that I was traveling to very distant parts of the world … during my dream journey the following canon occurred to me … As soon as I awoke, however, the canon had vanished and not one note of it could I recall. But on the following day as I was driving back here in the same vehicle, and was continuing yesterday's dream journey while awake, behold, in accordance with the law of the association of ideas, the same canon occurred to me.[12]

This letter, addressed to Tobias Haslinger, one of his publishers, includes the three-part canon inspired in his dream.

Although intelligence is a requirement for eminent creativity, there is no clear and close connection between the two: many intelligent individuals are not creative.[13] Intelligence is comprised of both verbal and nonverbal components and problem-solving is a key requirement. Although creative individuals make full use of a problem-solving capacity, they also require attributes such as application and motivation that are not related to intelligence. Lewis Terman (1877–1956) carried out extensive studies on the measurement of intelligence and its relation to giftedness; he also attempted to apply the principles of intelligence measurement to known historical "geniuses" such as British eugenicist Francis Galton (1822–1911). Terman's work was subsequently extended to a sample of 300 historically eminent men with very high abilities.[14] Cox estimated intelligence quotients (IQ) by using coded objective biographical and educational information. She found that the intelligence of these individuals was uniformly high, with the highest being that of Goethe, whose IQ was estimated to be 210; Beethoven's IQ was estimated to be 165. Cox also found that the ability to synthesize and to use practical techniques of communication and persuasion were important requirements for creativity.

A vivid imagination is essential for creativity as it enables the creative person to conceptualize an art form inwardly.[15] This representation may be purely ideational, or it may be verbal or auditory, depending on the tools and format of the art form. The individual must also possess the impetus, drive, and facilities to give concrete exterior form to the inner concept. Education and learning the "tools of the trade" are prerequisites to exteriorizing this concept. Developmental factors are vital to the genesis of creativity. Storr emphasizes the need for solitude, passivity, dependence, and even humility in the creative process.[16] Individuals who were creative as adults had often spent large parts of their childhood alone, due to separation, loss, or enforced isolation. He also notes that imaginative capacity is highly developed in creative individuals and that it is particularly active during childhood. Rothenberg found that identification and competition with the same-sex parent during early childhood influenced motivation toward the development of a career in the creative arts.[17]

Unusual childhood experiences can stimulate creativity. In a study of 699 eminent individuals, Eisenstadt found that parental loss by the age of ten was markedly greater among creative individuals than it was in the general population, and he concludes that the bereavement trauma enabled the child to assume increased responsibility, leading to the feeling that she or he was a "more worthwhile" person.[18] These difficulties translate into hard work and striving for achievement, accomplishment, and power, and a need to control her or his own destiny. Albert supports this conclusion and also finds that birth order was significant in eminent men; in a group of eminent individuals, forty-six percent were eldest sons, twenty percent were middle children, and fourteen percent were the youngest.[19] Albert uses his concept of the "special family position" to describe the situation where a gifted child is awarded a special role in the family and is guided toward success and achievement, a conclusion that has found more recent support.[20] Schubert, Wagner, and Schubert found that in a group of seventy-five composers of classical music, there was an over-representation of first-born sons.[21]

Many of these findings are relevant to Beethoven's situation. Since his older brother died in infancy, he became, in effect, the first-born son. He was gifted and had superior intellectual capacity. He also received special training in music and was strongly encouraged by his father and early teachers toward a career in music. His mother and young sister died when he was sixteen, but it is likely that the death of his grandfather, when Beethoven was three, was the major event in his psychological development. Although Beethoven had few actual memories of his grandfather, he had been named after him, was told many anecdotes about him during childhood, and kept his portrait with him throughout his life despite many changes of abode. Beethoven had all the characteristics of a child with a "special family position" to encourage and promote his career in music. He had the natural talent and the ego-strength to overcome the many setbacks he was forced to endure, such as the early deaths of his parents, grandfather, and two of his siblings, and he had the capacity to use these events to strengthen his confidence and autonomy and perfect his musical skills. Although he was not the "child prodigy" that Mozart had been at a comparable age, Beethoven nevertheless displayed exceptional talent and grew up in a social milieu that encouraged this talent to develop and mature.[22]

For creative art to have an impact on society it must be relevant to the social context of the period. This relevance may be present even if, at that particular point in history, the goals and vision of the artist are not synchronous with the goals and vision of the society in which he lives. Much creativity, even eminent creativity, goes unrecognized by society and emerges only after the death of the creator, sometimes generations later. For example, Copernicus' conclusion in the early sixteenth century that the sun, rather than the earth, was the centre of the solar system, brought him renown only after his death. The genius of Johann Sebastian Bach and Vincent van Gogh was recognized only after their deaths. Beethoven's talents were recognized while he was alive, and this recognition was facilitated by the fact that his music was concordant with the socio-political ethos of the era. The revolutionary nature of his compositions had resonance in the political revolutions that occurred during his lifetime.

More pragmatic motives may also spur an artist to create. Beethoven gave us at least three clues about his motives for composing: financial, spiritual, and health-related. He refers to the financial motive in letters on a number of occasions: "I am scrawling things for the sake of bread and money."[23] "It is hard to compose almost entirely for the sake of earning one's bread."[24] "Financial straits demand I compose every day."[25] In the Heiligenstadt Testament Beethoven describes deeper spiritual motives: "It seemed impossible to leave this world before I had produced all the works that I felt the urge to compose."[26] In 1823, he wrote to Schindler in the Conversation Books: "If I had to lose my vital force with life, what would have been left for the noble, the better."[27] The timing of this comment is relevant: Beethoven wrote it after recounting his lost love for Giulietta Guiccardi, saying that he might never have been able to compose the music he did had he married Guiccardi at the time of their romance. Another example of a spiritual motive appears in a letter to the publishing firm Bernard Schotts Söhne: "Apollo and the Muses are not yet going to let me be handed over to Death, for I still owe them much; and before my departure for the Elysian fields, I must leave behind me what the Eternal Spirit has infused into my soul and bids me complete. Why, I feel as if I had hardly composed more than few notes."[28] Finally, Beethoven's creativity was also spurred on by health-related issues. In a note to Anton Schindler in the Conversation Books in 1825 he writes: "My doctor saved me, because I could no longer write music [his eyes were bothering him at the time], but now I can write notes which help to relieve me of my troubles."[29]

Louis Schlosser (1800–1886), a musician and composer, gives a penetrating description of Beethoven's compositional process. During a meeting with Beethoven in 1823, he reported the composer as saying:

I carry my thoughts about with me for a long time, sometimes a very long time, before I set them down. At the same time my memory is so faithful to me that I am sure not to forget a theme which I have once conceived even after years have passed. I make many changes, reject and reattempt until I am satisfied. Then the working out in breadth, length, height and depth begins in my head, and since

I am conscious of what I want, the basic idea never leaves me. It rises, grows upward, and I hear and see the picture as a whole take shape and stand forth before me as though cast in a single piece, so that all that is left is the work of writing it down. This goes quickly, according as I have the time, for sometimes I have several compositions in labour at once, though I am sure never to confuse one with the other. You will ask me whence I take my ideas? That I cannot say with any degree of certainty: they come to me uninvited, directly or indirectly. I could almost grasp them in my hands, out in Nature's open, in the woods, during my promenades, in the silence of the night, at earliest dawn. They are roused by moods which in the poet's case are transmuted into words and in mine into tones, that sound, roar and storm until at last they take shape for me as notes.[30]

Schindler also describes the drama and passion that Beethoven could experience when composing [at the time he was working on the *Missa Solemnis*].

From behind the closed door of one of the parlours we could hear the master working on the fugue of the Credo, singing, yelling, stamping his feet. When we had heard enough of this almost frightening performance, and were about to depart, the door opened and Beethoven stood before us, his features distorted to the point of inspiring terror. He looked as though he had just engaged in a life and death struggle with a whole army of contrapuntists, his everlasting enemies.[31]

These examples indicate that Beethoven had both material and deeper spiritual motives for composing. We know from his biography and his character that he was a lonely and self-centered – but also self-sufficient – man, and that he had a powerful inner compulsion to externalize his musical ideas, even when he experienced deep personal restraints related to his emotions, his health, or external barriers caused by rejection or conflicts with others.

What role does brain structure and function play in musical creativity? As a result of major advances in technology, the last fifteen years have witnessed a burgeoning interest in the neurobiology of this topic. Complex diagnostic instruments such as the PET (positive emission tomography) scans, the functional MRI (magnetic resonance imaging), and magneto-encephalography are sensitive to neuronal activity and have been used to identify localized areas of brain function in response to a wide variety of musical stimuli. For example, dissonance and changes in pitch and rhythm have been used as stimuli, and responses have been compared for different groups such as professional musicians versus non-musicians, children versus adults, and individuals with congenital amusia (tone deafness) versus those without this condition. Although the results of such testing are not always consistent, they have shown that brain function in response to musical stimuli changes with age, musical sophistication, and the presence of certain brain lesions. More remarkably, the emotional effects of music are mediated by the same areas of the brain that are implicated in other emotional stimuli.[32] Zatore concludes that music activates the areas of the brain that are essential for evolutionary survival – the nucleus accumbens, the dorsal midbrain, and the insula – even though music itself is not essential. In studies of individuals with congenital amusia, Peretz concludes that the human brain has neural networks that are specific to the processing of music[33] and suggests that music has biological roots, that it is not just a cultural artifact, and that it serves needs that are so important that the brain dedicates neural space to its processing.

An interaction between music and the brain has also been found in certain neurological conditions. Brust found that brain disease could affect or be affected by music either positively or negatively.[34] For example, certain musical sounds could provoke seizures or hallucinations in some individuals and a neurological disease could affect the appreciation of pitch or rhythm. Brust provides several clinical examples from the literature, including the composer Maurice Ravel, who developed a progressive neurological disease that included aphasia, agraphia, and apraxia: he was still able to listen to music critically but he lost the ability to compose. Creativity, artistic imagery, and musical appreciation have traditionally been linked with the activity and function of the right hemisphere, whereas the left is concerned with cognition, language, and the organization of intellectual faculties.[35] Other researchers in this field have concluded that although there is an association between music and neuronal responsiveness in the right cerebral hemisphere, musical processing is widely distributed through both hemispheres and the full integrity of the whole brain is a requirement for eminent creativity.[36]

Psychological research has shown that eminent creativity requires an end product that is both useful and original, and this end product must have wide social acceptance. Social and developmental factors such as family relationships and the "special family position" of a child are important in facilitating later creativity. The personal traits of intelligence, imagination, application, and motivation are essential prerequisites, and motivation, in turn, is affected by the compulsion to exteriorize a vivid inner experience. Beethoven's life provides eloquent expression for each of these elements.

PSYCHOPATHOLOGY AND CREATIVITY

Psychopathology, substance dependency (including alcoholism), and medical health problems can affect creativity. "Psychopathology" is a general term that denotes the different forms and patterns of mental illness. Many anecdotal reports and some scientific research have supported a relationship between creativity and psychological maladjustment. A longstanding belief that genius and "madness" are linked can be traced back to Aristotle, who describes a connection between genius and melancholy.[37] Shakespeare phrases this belief succinctly: "The lunatic, the lover, and the poet, Are of imagination all compact" (*A Midsummer Night's Dream*, V.i.7). Belief in the creativity–madness connection became widespread during the nineteenth century. French writer Louis-François Lelut, a strong proponent of this connection, was supported in England by Francis Galton among others. However, many eminent individuals opposed this viewpoint, including George Bernard Shaw in England and American psychologist Lewis Terman.[38] Debate about this connection became almost farcical when Emile Zola submitted himself to examination – ostensibly in the interests of science – by a group of psychiatrists led by Dr Toulouse, head of the faculty of medicine in Paris:[39] their report, published with Zola's approval, concludes that Zola was "neurotic" (*névro-*

pathe) and that his nervous system was excitable and unusually sensitive (*douloureux*). Zola, at least, was proud of his reputation of being both creative and "mad." In the mid-1970s Becker noted that the number of writers supporting this association gradually diminished and had virtually disappeared by the mid-twentieth century. Becker believed that the supporting evidence was false and had been promoted by a romantic notion of the association between madness, the supernatural, and genius.[40] In this context, it is highly regrettable that Becker and others have used the inappropriate and emotive term "madness" in their works. This term is pejorative and has no place in contemporary discussion of this topic; the allusion applies also to the word "lunatic" used by Shakespeare in the quotation above.

There are many anecdotal examples illustrating the connection between creativity and psychopathology. Robert Schumann, Pyotr Il'yich Tchaikovsky, Vincent van Gogh, and Ernest Hemingway are all famous men of art who suffered from severe depressions that led to their early deaths from direct or indirect suicide. The composer Robert Schumann almost certainly suffered from bipolar disorder (the coexistence of both depression and hypomanic swings of mood)[41] and he may also have had syphilis.[42] Slater and Meyer note that Schumann's musical productivity was much increased in 1840 and 1849, both years in which his mood was consistently elevated throughout the year; conversely, his output was reduced during his "depressed" years. A specific connection between mood and creativity is found in the writings of American poet Emily Dickinson.[43] Analysis of her poems shows not only frequent themes of depression and suicidality but also "seasonality" – she did much of her writing during the summer months and relatively little in the winter – and her correspondence reflects both gloom and elation. In a commentary on McDermott's paper about Emily Dickinson, Kalian and his colleagues concede that there are difficulties in making post-mortem psychiatric diagnoses.[44] In a study of writings by Nikolai Gogol, the nineteenth-century Russian author, despite their stated reservations about post-mortem diagnoses they found a close correlation between the quality and quantity of his writing on the one hand and his changes of mood as discerned in his diaries and letters on the other: they conclude that he likely had bipolar disorder.

Over the last thirty years a substantial volume of experimental research has accumulated to show that the connection between genius and illness is more than just anecdotal or coincidental.[45] Prentky concluded that the cognitive styles of highly creative individuals "bore a striking resemblance to psychotic-like thinking ... the cognitive flexibility necessary to realize extraordinary conceptual insights and theoretical breakthroughs is characteristic, in a less severe form, of psychotic thought process."[46] He also studied the social context in which the creativity occurred and makes the perceptive observation that anguish and despair derived from external civil disturbances might be a source of inspiration to creative artists. The example he gives is the period of prolific creativity and widespread appreciation of the arts in Tsarist Russia during the late nineteenth century, a setting of social and political turmoil.[47] Another example of a rich flowering of creativity in a climate of social and political anguish is the literature, art, and music that flourished in the restrictive regime of apartheid South Africa during the second half of the twentieth century. Music, including singing and dance, helped spur resistance to apartheid and provided a cohesive and rallying force for activists, particularly those in prison.

In his extensive and scholarly review of this field, Eysenck concludes that the balance of evidence favours an association between creativity and psychopathology.[48] He postulates a personality trait that he calls "psychoticism," which he defines as a temperamental disposition rendering an individual more likely to develop a psychosis. He considers that "overinclusiveness" – the exaggerated tendency to verbally express a variety of interconnected ideas – is a characteristic of both psychopathology and creativity.[49] The traits characteristic of psychoticism include aggressiveness, impulsivity, coldness, egocentricity, and tough-mindedness. This last feature, analogous to "ego strength" (personal power and strength of character), enables the creative individual to triumph over real and perceived adversity and rejection, and to overcome or at least channel even the tendency to mental illness. Eysenck's many examples of geniuses who have shown these characteristics include Max Planck, William Harvey,

Louis Pasteur, and Isaac Newton. It is clear from Beethoven's life and character that he likely had traits of psychoticism but was able to use his ego strength to battle against internal and external demons and overcame them because of an inner conviction of the power of his message.

In a highly original survey D.K. Simonton[50] found a statistical link between "stress" and musical creativity. Simonton studied the musical productivity – judged according to the quality and quantity of creative output during successive five-year blocks – of ten well-known male composers: Bach, Beethoven, Mozart, Haydn, Brahms, Handel, Debussy, Schubert, Wagner, and Chopin. In his analysis, which included the effects of age, physical illness, social reinforcement, stress, war intensity, and internal (civil) disturbances, he found that the more works a composer produced; the more likely some of these works were to be considered "major" rather than "minor." As might be expected, physical illness had an adverse effect on the number of compositions composed in a given five-year block, but stress, war intensity, civil disturbances, and social reinforcement had no apparent connection with productivity. Although Simonton was not concerned with psychopathology per se, he concludes that musical creativity persists no matter what the environment provided in terms of rewards, anxieties, and distractions: creativity is driven more by intrinsic than by extrinsic factors. In a well-designed study Nancy Andreason and her colleagues found a link between creativity and affective disorder.[51] Using a structured diagnostic interview, Andreason assessed twenty-seven male and three female writers, and a comparable control group of non-writers. Results showed that while none of the writers' group suffered from schizophrenia, both mood disorders and alcoholism were significantly more prevalent in the writer group than in the control group. Andreason explains this difference by suggesting that affective disorder provides some cultural advantages to society.

Felix Post used a different method of exploring this connection in a wide-ranging article on psychopathology in eminent historical figures.[52] Post carefully read the biographies of 291 highly creative individuals who had been born and died between 1830 and 1980 (so unfortunately Beethoven was not included). Post divided the list of these individuals, all of whom were judged to have achieved lasting international fame in their chosen fields, into six groups: visual artists (48), thinkers (50), scientists (45), statesmen (46), composers (52), and novelists (50). He then made a psychiatric diagnosis of each individual – according to the DSM-III-R diagnostic system – based on the biographical material (including medical reports but not the biographer's interpretation of these reports). A distinction corresponding to the Axis I and Axis II categories of DSM-III-R was made between episodic disorders (psychiatric illnesses) and lifelong psychopathology (deviations of personality), and the psychopathology of each individual was assigned a category according to level of severity: none, mild, moderate, or severe. Analysis of the results showed that scientists had the lowest prevalence of severe psychopathology (17.8%) and that the rate increased steadily through composers, politicians, artists, and thinkers, with the highest prevalence present in writers (46%). With reference to personality disorder, traits such as anxiety, dependency, and obsessionality were predominant and were found in 38.9% of the sample, with relatively little difference between the six groups. "Severe" episodic psychiatric disorders – sufficient to interfere with function, daily life, and relationships – occurred in an average of 27% of the total group, with the highest level found in writers (42%) and the lowest in politicians (21.7%). Depression and alcoholism were most prevalent in writers and less so in artists and composers. Of the total group, 11% had alcohol dependence. The fact that schizophrenia was unusual, affecting only 1% of the total group, which is also its prevalence in the general population, argues against a link between schizophrenia and creativity. From this report Post concluded that there was a "causal nexus" between psychopathology and creativity and that depression and alcoholism had higher-than-expected prevalence rates, particularly in writers and artists. He did not speculate what this causal nexus might be, or why prevalence rates were higher in writers as compared to other artistic groups. A more recent study of forty American jazz musicians confirmed a connection between psychopathology and creativity.[53]

Although Beethoven was not in the group of composers studied by Post, it is clear that the method of analysis described in this volume – using biographical material to assess and interpret Beethoven's medical and psychiatric problems – is similar to that used by Post. Using his criteria to assess severity of psychopathology, Beethoven would rank as being at least in the "moderately severe" category: he became suicidally depressed at times, and this led to serious disruptions in his interpersonal relationships, but the depressed episodes did not affect his compositional capacity in an enduring manner, nor did he require the equivalent of what now would be called hospital treatment. Using similar methods, A.M. Ludwig assessed 1,000 individuals in the United States who had high levels of creative achievement. He found similar results to Post's,[54] and showed that those in the creative arts had a higher rate of alcohol-related problems, depression, mania, and psychosis; they also had more therapy than the other subgroups. Public officials, military men, businessmen, and social and physical scientists formed the most "stable" categories. Ludwig concluded that the creative arts might attract predisposed individuals, and that certain stressors peculiar to the arts might aggravate their difficulties. Ludwig also considered that these professions might foster certain forms of psychopathology, such as might be expressed by extreme forms of extroversion, as a vehicle to success. The higher levels of psychopathology might relate also to the impersonal, non-stylistic, and public nature of careers in the arts.

Another study found a high prevalence of both depression and alcoholism in a group of fifteen abstract expressionist artists.[55] Seven of the artists died before age sixty (two from suicide and two from single-car accidents), a proportion much higher than that of a comparable sample of the general population. The researchers postulate that the mental depression of the artists might be creatively adaptive, since it helped to bring spiritual values into focus in a secular and materialistic age. An editorial commentary on this paper debates whether treatment of a creative artist with depression or bipolar disorder would help or hinder creativity[56] and concludes that if the illness was severe, the creative process would be improved by treatment. This result is borne out by Schou, who treated twenty-four artists with manic-depressive illness: he found that in twelve of the artists, creativity was improved on lithium, in six it had no effect, and in six creativity diminished.[57] In a thought-provoking aside, Schou notes that several of those whose creativity was reduced chose to stop the medication, preferring to be "manic" and creative, rather than unproductive.

Kay Jamison's engrossing book *Touched with Fire* presents forceful arguments favouring the association between creativity and psychopathology.[58] She provides numerous examples of the prevalence of psychopathology in creative individuals and states that the main purpose of her book is to make the case for "the compelling association between the artistic and the manic-depressive temperament." Jamison lists thirty-five English poets, only eight of whom had no indication of psychiatric disorder,[59] and notes that the list of writers and artists who ended their lives by suicide is "staggeringly long."[60] Jamison also provides a list of the many poets, writers, and composers who had probable cyclothymia or manic-depressive illness,[61] and she considers milder forms of hypomania as representing the productive phases of the illness.[62]

H. Bower puts forward the provocative suggestion that Beethoven suffered from a "creative illness" between 1815 and 1820.[63] Creative illness is a concept developed by Henri Ellenberger, who describes it as a severe neurotic or sometimes even psychotic condition in which a creative individual is obsessed by the pursuit of some difficult aim:[64] for a period of three years or more, the artist feels isolated and unproductive, and struggles with attempts at self-healing; recovery, when it occurs, is spontaneous and rapid and is accompanied by euphoria and a transformation of personality – the individual feels as if she or he had gained access to a new spiritual world, and the illness was followed by a burst of creativity. Ellenberger's examples of individuals who experienced this condition include Robert Burton (1577–1640), George Cheyne (1671–1743), Sigmund Freud (1856–1939), Pierre Janet (1859–1947), and Carl Gustav Jung (1875–1961). A review of Beethoven's life between 1812 and 1817 reveals that many of his experiences fit the description of a creative illness. He was unproductive, at least until 1817, he had a number of medical and psychiatric problems,[65] and his "recovery," when it occurred, was followed by his mature and final period, which opened up a whole new dimension in musical composition, in which spirituality played a key role. The concept of creative illness merits further examination, not only in Beethoven's situation but in the lives of other creative individuals as well.

To explain why there appears to be an association between manic-depressive disorder and creativity is a more difficult task. Although speculative, there are a number of possibilities to consider. The connection could be genetic. Manic-depressive disorder is known to have a strong genetic component, and there is likely a genetic component to creativity as well. It would therefore be possible for both the disorder and a creative capacity to arise from a common gene or genetic combination. Research arising from the Human Genome Project may ultimately provide an answer to this question. The connection could also be phenomenological, that is, related to the particular characteristics of those mental conditions related to creativity. Bipolar disorder is a condition that affects thought, mood, and behaviour, and the way in which thought process is affected may have a special relevance to creativity. R.A. Prentky notes the importance of "cognitive flexibility" – a concept analogous to the phrase "lateral thinking" used by other writers – in creativity.[66] These terms describe a type of thinking characterized by the capacity to "move sideways" (as a knight does on a chessboard), rather than in a simple, straightforward, linear fashion. This process of thinking stimulates originality and novel ideas, and when focused and purposeful, it is a key feature of creative endeavour.

It is not coincidental that this type of thinking is also characteristic of "flights of ideas" or "racing thoughts" found in people with hypomania. Their thought process, as expressed in speech, flits from one topic to another, although there is an underlying theme that makes it appear cohesive and appropriate. Such individuals are full of drive and energy. They set goals, work intensively toward these goals, and often make do with less sleep than the average person. They may also be over-confident and expansive, and although irritability is a common feature, this does not necessarily deflect them from striving to attain their self-set goals. Efficiency and goal-directed function are affected only if the condition becomes more severe. Hypomania is often associated with a feeling of euphoria, which acts as a further spur to purposeful activity. Many patients with this condition have pleaded *not* to have treatment because they revelled in their elated state of mind.

The rarity of schizophrenia among creative individuals has been noted above. However MacGregor described three artists who had schizophrenia – F.-X. Messerschmidt (1736–1783), John Martin (1782–1838), and James Matthews (early nineteenth century) – and depicts the bizarre effect that their mental states had on their art.[67] No eminent composer is known to have suffered from schizophrenia.

Manic-depressive disorder is distinct from schizophrenia in that manic-depression is, by definition, phasic or recurrent. Between episodes, therefore, the individual is left healthy and functioning for extended periods of time. The statement that there is an association between psychopathology (particularly manic-depression) and creativity is an affirmation that creativity may be enhanced or stimulated while an individual is suffering from milder forms of these conditions. This does not mean that the individual is creative *because* he or she suffers from these conditions. Moreover, it is likely that creativity can be maintained during all phases of manic-depression, as long as the condition is not severe.

When we apply this data to Beethoven, we find that he was able to continue composing even when depressed. For example, he was likely very depressed when he wrote the Heiligenstadt Testament in 1802, but during this period he was composing, among other works, the second and third symphonies (op. 36 and op. 55) and the set of three piano sonatas, op. 31. With the exception of the *Marche funèbre* in the Symphony no. 3 ("Eroica"), none of these compositions are depressing. Indeed, the final movement of the third symphony is optimistic and exuberant. The likely explanation for this paradox is that Beethoven was sublimating his depressive symptoms through intensive composition. The fact that many of these works have a positive and optimistic quality also indicates that he was overcompensating for his sadness – that is, writing music that expressed, in an exaggerated form, the opposite feeling to his state of mind and mood at the time. Composition of such music helped him to "work through" and heal, at least for a time, his emotions and his depression. For Beethoven, therefore, composing was therapeutic.

Beethoven's hypomanic episodes (if that is what they were) were brief and self-limiting, and did not have an adverse effect on his creativity; indeed, they likely promoted it, as is suggested by this review. He was also helped by personality traits such as the capacity to remain focused on goals, the painstaking care with which he recorded and developed his musical ideas, and his musical "perfectionism." He had the capacity to compose several different works simultaneously, and even if he put one aside temporarily, he could return to it and pick up the theme and relevant ideas in a short space of time. With major large-scale works such as the Ninth Symphony and the *Missa Solemnis*, Beethoven had the patience and the application to work on musical ideas for years to bring them to fruition.

What effect does psychopathology have on the content, subject matter, and quality of the created work? The expectation is that mental depression would lead to the creation of gloomy and foreboding works, and this indeed appears often to be the case. The deeply introspective quality of Beethoven's music written during his third and final periods has been noted above. In 1802, with the dawning awareness of the development of his deafness, he was composing the Eroica Symphony. This work, and indeed much of his later music, has sudden and changing contrasts of musical mood that are consistent with the frequent and sudden changes of emotional mood that characterized his behaviour at that time. Beethoven expresses musical anger in *Rondo a capriccio*, op. 129, a whimsical piece that has come to be known as "The Rage over a Lost Penny." In her analysis of Beethoven's String Quartet in B flat major, op. 18, no. 6, (*La malincola*), Caldwell notes the six alternating slow and fast sections and a phasic quality that describes, in musical terms, the fluctuations of mood and activity that occur in the cyclothymic temperament,[68] and she concludes: "This is the only [musical] composition that has made a psychiatric term immortal." (This is not quite accurate if we remember that "rage" can also be considered, in some respects, a psychiatric term.) Although a detailed analysis of the relationship between Beethoven's moods and his compositions has not been carried out, these examples illustrate the ways in which his music reflected his emotions, feelings, and behaviour. A relationship between mood and the subject matter of creativity can be discerned also in other artists. For example, Mozart was in the midst of composing a *Requiem* (funeral mass) in the weeks leading up to his death.[69] In the days leading up to his suicide, Van Gogh painted fields of corn with roads leading nowhere, the whole covered by dark, angry-looking clouds.[70] Brahms developed cancer six months before his death, and knowing that he was dying (even though he did not want to know), he wrote eleven neo-Baroque chorale preludes for organ, including the wistful *O Welt, ich muss dich lassen* (O World, I must leave thee).[71]

The traditional belief that creativity is linked to psychopathology is thus verified by more recent scientific research. Depression, bipolar disorder, and suicide all have a high prevalence among creative artists. This connection is a statistical one: as a group, creative artists are more likely to have these conditions than are non-creative people. Many, likely the majority, of creative individuals are unaffected. Further, this association applies only to mild or moderate forms of psychopathology. Severe illness thwarts creativity, at least during the period that the illness is acute.[72]

SUBSTANCE ABUSE AND CREATIVITY

There is much anecdotal evidence that the prevalence of substance abuse among creative artists, writers, and musicians is high. Alcohol is the most common substance because of its ready availability, but drug abuse (both of medically prescribed and non-medical drugs) also occurs. Rothenberg[73] studied the biographies of thirty highly creative individuals, mainly writers, all of whom had problems of excess alcohol use, including such well-known names as Charles Baudelaire, Louise Bogan, Truman Capote, John Cheever, F. Scott Fitzgerald, Ernest Hemingway, Victor Hugo, James Joyce, O. Henry, John Steinbeck, Dylan Thomas, and Tennessee Williams. Rothenberg found little evidence that these creative people wrote while under the influence of alcohol, but he considered that Hemingway, Fitzgerald, and O. Henry might have used alcohol to stimulate their creativity. Rothenberg, who was a psychiatrist, also describes parts of his treatment of John Cheever, whom he encouraged to join Alcoholics Anonymous in order to control his drinking, and states that writers might use alcohol to cope with the anxiety generated by the creative process. To the above list we can add other men of art who had alcohol problems: artists Henri Toulouse-Lautrec, Paul Gauguin, and probably Vincent van Gogh (at least during his Paris period); musicians Pyotr Tchaikovsky, Modest Mussorgsky, Nikolai Rimsky-Korsakov, and Eric Satie; and poets W.H. Auden and Samuel Coleridge. A biographer of Tchaikovsky notes that he would sit in restaurants until three o'clock in the morning, that he could drink a great deal of wine yet keep his full mental powers, and that very few of his friends could keep up with him in this respect.[74] Satie suffered from frequent hangovers: a colleague had to bolt Satie in his room during the afternoon in order to stop him from drinking so that he would be able to perform at the cabarets in the evening.[75] An in-depth survey of fifteen modern artists found that five had serious alcohol abuse problems, a proportion substantially higher than would be expected from population studies where the lifetime prevalence of alcoholism is approximately twenty percent.[76] However, a number of additional factors, including age, heredity, health, and socioeconomic status also affect the pattern and prevalence of alcoholism in particular individuals or groups.

In his study of eminent historical individuals Post made diagnoses of alcoholism in 29.2% of the artists, 28% of the writers, and 21.2% of the composers – but he did not have a comparable control group.[77] The lower percentages in the remaining groups explains why the average for the whole group was only 11.7%. In her assessment of writers Andreason found that the prevalence of substance dependency was much higher among the creative than the non-creative group (30% versus 7%) when the two groups were matched for socioeconomic status.[78]

At first sight, it may appear puzzling that creativity can coexist with alcohol abuse. Alcohol is a central nervous system depressant, and when taken in large quantities over an extended period, it is toxic to the brain, causing such syndromes as hallucinosis, paranoia, delirium tremens, Korsakov's psychosis, Wernicke's encephalopathy, and, at the final stage, dementia. With the exception of the latter two conditions, these syndromes are largely reversible, providing that the alcohol intake is stopped. Over-indulgence in alcohol (alcohol "dependence" as distinct from "abuse"; see chapter 4 for a more detailed discussion of these conditions) does not generally result in these neuropsychiatric syndromes but can nevertheless affect other systems of the body such as the liver, blood, heart, and stomach, apart from its many social and legal consequences. Although alcohol is a central nervous system depressant, it affects different brain levels at a variable time/dose sequence. The higher centres of the brain – in particular the parts responsible for judgment, decision-making, and social control of behaviour – are affected earliest and most severely following the intake of alcohol. It is for this reason that people "under the influence" become disinhibited, lose self-control, and perform actions and behaviours that are out of character.

But can alcohol actually promote the creative impulse? It is possible that creativity is released, at least in part, by the disinhibiting effect of alcohol, and biographers provide many examples of this among creative individuals. Mussorgsky's final years, despite his drinking, were described not as a decline but as a rebirth.[79] Toulouse-Lautrec continued to paint even when his life had sunk into debauchery and dipsomania, and "far from clouding his brain, drinking sharpened it."[80] Tchaikovsky drank large quantities of alcohol into the small hours of the morning, yet was able to retain his mental powers.[81] Auden's poems written when he was not under the influence of alcohol exhibit an uncharacteristic "flatness of tone."[82] "Alcohol has the power to stimulate the mystical faculties of human nature," wrote William James in 1902.[83] Coleridge's wonderful poem *Kubla Khan*, written when he was under the influence of opium, is an example of the use of a drug other than alcohol for creative purposes.[84] The key to explaining how alcohol or some drugs may stimulate creativity, therefore, appears to be that enough must be taken to disinhibit the higher brain centres, but not so much that the whole central nervous system is inactivated.

One of the few experimental studies on this topic looks at the effects of alcohol on creativity in a group of psychology students.[85] Creative thinking was measured using a specially designed test, and results were compared between two groups, one of which had received alcohol. The administration of alcohol was disguised by tonic, so that those who received it were not aware that they were being given alcohol. Results showed that both groups performed equally well. The major difference between the two groups was that those who believed that they received alcohol rated their performance significantly more favourably than those who believed they had received only the tonic placebo. The authors conclude that people apply more lenient standards to evaluating their performance when they believe they have been drinking, and that the cognitive changes induced by alcohol enable them to dismiss perfectionism and rely on instinct to facilitate initiation, maintenance, and enjoyment of the creative process. Although this experiment can be regarded as an artificial and perhaps even simplistic survey, the results were unexpected and suggest that the relationship between drinking alcohol and creativity is more complex than it appears on the surface.

These conclusions should not be used to justify using alcohol to stimulate creativity. Alcohol is a health hazard when taken in anything more than small quantities. However the overuse of alcohol does not in itself kill the creative impulse, and in certain individuals at certain times, it may promote it. Returning to Beethoven, the prevalence of alcohol problems among artists indicate that there is no reason why he could not have continued to create the musical wonders of his final years, even though he was taking alcohol in sufficient quantity to seriously impair his liver function and hasten his demise. At times the alcohol may even have assisted him, by providing a self-administered "tranquilizing" agent that vicariously enabled him to cope with, or at least better tolerate, the traumatic events of the final twelve years of his life.

MEDICAL ILLNESS AND CREATIVITY

There are many examples of serious illnesses affecting the quality of an artist's work. Until the mid-twentieth century, tuberculosis was a common, chronic, and potentially fatal illness that was associated with overcrowding and poor socio-economic circumstances. There has also been a recent and unexpected increase in prevalence, even in developed countries. Thomas Mann's superb novel *The Magic Mountain* is based on his experiences in a tuberculosis sanatorium. George Orwell knew that he was dying of tuberculosis and hastened to complete his novel *Nineteen Eighty-Four*; his awareness of approaching death "heightened his emotions and powers of expression."[86] Winston Smith, the chief character in this futuristic tale, is Orwell's last, gloomy self-portrait. Frédéric Chopin, on the other hand, became depressed and listless when he realized that his death from tuberculosis was near; his will to compose almost deserted him, and his last composition, the Mazurka in F minor, op. 68, no. 4, expresses "deathly weariness."[87] It is thought that Mozart likely died during an attack of acute rheumatic fever, although his death may have been precipitated by bleeding therapy to which he was subjected.[88] During his final few weeks he was able to work intermittently on the *Requiem*, which was never completed, although brief rehearsals were held in his sick room.[89] Jane Austen had Addison's Disease (a depletion of the hormones secreted by the adrenal medulla gland, and often the result of tuberculosis), which caused her to feel listless and dull and affected her bodily functions but not her mind. She overcame these feelings to complete her final novel, *Persuasion*, which was published posthumously.[90]

In a report on the "swan song phenomenon" – the effect on musical composition of a composer's perception of approaching death – in 172 composers, Simonton found that physical illness had an adverse effect on musical creativity.[91] Simonton's methodology was complex and incorporated variables of melodic originality, repertoire popularity, aesthetic significance, and listener accessibility. He concludes that career swan songs were brief and relatively simple in melodic structure, but profound enough to secure a lasting place in the concert hall. The swan song was "an expression of resignation and contentment, rather than despair or tragedy." Post briefly considered physical health in his examination of 291 highly creative individuals and found that cardiac and cerebral atherosclerosis were the commonest cause of death, with infections ranking second.[92] Average age at death was highest among scientists and thinkers and lowest among composers. Post himself does not draw any inferences from these findings.

A number of writers have studied the effects of deafness in musicians. Hood notes that in addition to Beethoven, Bedřich Smetana, Ralph Vaughan Williams, and Gabriel Fauré became deaf during their composing lives.[93] Smetana was totally deaf by age fifty-six; at a piano recital given in his honour, he "played with such originality, feeling and expression ... that many wept for his fate."[94] After composing a series of orchestral and operatic works, Smetana stated, "I never heard a note of all these works and still they lived on in me, and through mental imagery alone moved me to tears and sheer ecstasy." Vaughan Williams became deaf in his seventies. Although he could not hear high tones, he continued conducting with the use of an ear trumpet, which he preferred to a hearing aid. His widow wrote, "He had a lifetime knowledge of various works ... experience in both writing and conducting music ... knowledge and expectation of what should be there filled gaps in music and imagination."[95] In discussing Beethoven's deafness, Hood suggests that it may have been "sensorineural" in type (that is, the result of disease of the auditory nerve) and that it was caused by an earlier attack of typhus fever. As noted above, however, there is no certainty that Beethoven ever had typhus fever, and the fact that he was able to hear vibration is not consistent with disease of the auditory nerve. Hood concludes: "The supreme paradox is that, of all those afflicted with the catastrophe of deafness, the composer is the best equipped to bear it because he alone can revert to and find satisfaction and fulfillment in his own musical imagery. In his mind he can create perfection."[96] Beethoven was thus able to turn the defeat of deafness into the victory of written music.[97]

Beethoven had unpleasant and chronic health problems for most of his life. Although he complained frequently and bitterly about them, he also dealt with them in a stoic fashion, and he rarely let them interfere with his composing. This is true particularly of his hearing problem. Although it caused him immense grief, and brought him to the point of suicide in 1802, he dealt with it by slowly letting go of teaching, conducting, and performing (in all of which he was limited by his hearing defect), and focused his musical energies increasingly, and during his final years solely, on composition, which he could master without hearing. This channeling of his creative energy into composing may, by this very fact alone, have raised the fineness and the quality of his works and enabled him to better deal with the anguish of his deafness. It forced him to search deep inside himself for new harmonic and structural possibilities to produce original musical effects. This could only have happened, of course, if he had the innate genius, drive, and theoretical knowledge gained from the intensive musical education of his formative years. He knew and understood musical notation, its meaning, interpretation, and sound effect consequences. Both nature and nurture were developed to a high degree, and, as Beethoven stated himself, his main motive to compose was the need to express and externalize this inner urge.

We can never understand all the reasons for Beethoven's creativity. He came to maturity at a critical time in political and musical history, and because of his natural talent he was able to ride the crests of both these waves. In the final analysis, he possessed, probably like all those touched by the highest levels of creativity, an indefinable inner impulse that demanded expression, even in the face of seemingly impassable internal and external barriers. He possessed and expressed to the highest degree that intangible and ineffable quality that humankind shares with its Creator.

APPENDICES

Glossary of Medical Terms

This glossary was developed with the assistance of Dorland's *Illustrated Medical Dictionary*, 29th ed. (Philadelphia: Saunders, 2000), and the *Oxford English Dictionary*, compact edition (New York: Oxford University Press, 1982).

acne: A chronic inflammatory disease of the sebaceous glands in the skin that most commonly affects the face, chest, and back. Also called common acne or acne vulgaris.

Affective Disorder: A group of mental disorders, the essential feature of which is a disturbance of mood with one or more episodes of depression or mania, or some combination of these mood changes.

Agraphia: Loss of the ability to write.

Amusia: Loss of the ability to recognize musical pitch; sometimes called "tone-deafness."

anaemia: A reduction below normal in the concentration of the red blood corpuscles or the hemoglobin in the blood that occurs when the equilibrium between blood loss (through bleeding or destruction) and blood production is disturbed.

anti-lithic: An agent that prevents the formation of a stone or calculus.

aphasia: Loss of the ability to speak.

apraxia: Loss of the ability to carry out familiar movements despite the absence of muscle weakness.

asthma: Recurrent attacks of shortness of breath accompanied by inflammation or wheezing due to contraction of the smaller bronchial tubes of the lungs.

auditory nerve: The eighth cranial nerve that connects the inner ear with the brain. It transmits information to the brain about sound, and about position, balance, and movement.

aural cartilage: The internal plate of elastic cartilage that is found in the external ear; also called the auricular cartilage.

auricular artery: A small artery supplying the inner and middle ear with oxygen and nutrients.

bed sore: An ulceration of the skin caused by prolonged pressure in a patient allowed to lie too still in bed for a long period of time; also called a pressure or a decubitus sore or ulcer.

bile duct: The channel between the gall bladder and the upper part of the small intestine that enters the intestine at the same point as the duct from the pancreas. The bile duct transports enzymes and other biochemicals produced in the liver to the intestine.

biliary gravel: The term applied to the fairly coarse concretions of mineral salts that are of smaller than so called "stones," that may be found in gall bladder and bile duct.

bipolar disorder: A type of mood disorder in which both depressive and hypomanic or manic episodes occur; also called manic-depressive disorder.

bronchitis: Inflammation of a bronchus or bronchi (the channels that carry air, and connect the trachea to the air sacs in the periphery of the lungs).

calyx: Cup-shaped organs in the kidneys that collect the urine before it passes down into the bladder.

capillaries: Microscopic blood vessels that connect the small arteries (flowing away from the heart) with the small veins (flowing back to the heart) completing the circulation of the blood.

catarrh: Inflammation of a mucous membrane with the free discharge of mucous; generally applied to the upper respiratory tract.

cathartics: Agents that cause emptying of the bowels.

cirrhosis: A disease of the liver in which cells are replaced by non-functioning fibrous tissue. There are a number of possible causes; during the nineteenth century the most common cause was the chronic ingestion of excessive quantities of alcohol.

cochlea: A spirally wound tube resembling a snail shell that forms part of the inner ear.

colic: Acute abdominal pain that fluctuates, often widely, in severity.

concha: The hollow of the auricle of the external ear.

conversion disorder: A psychiatric condition characterized by a physical symptom, and caused by the transformation of inner anxiety or conflict into a somatic manifestation.

cow pox: A mild, self-limited skin disease caused by a virus that affects the udders of milk cows; it can also infect the milkers, causing a rash on the hands and fingers.

cupping: The operation of drawing blood by scarifying the skin, and applying a cupping glass, the air in which is then rarified.

delirium tremens: An acute medical condition characterized by agitation, hallucinations, illusions, delusions, and other symptoms, and caused by the sudden cessation of drinking in a person used to taking large quantities of alcohol over an extended period.

dementia: A medical condition characterized by the gradual, and usually progressive loss of intellectual functions such as memory, concentration, abstract thinking, and other cognitive functions.

diabetes mellitus: A disorder of carbohydrate metabolism, caused by a failure of the pancreas to produce the hormone insulin. The resulting metabolic malfunctions can affect many organs in the body and are fatal if the insulin is not replaced.

diaphoretics: Agents that promote sweating.

diarrhea: Abnormal frequency of bowel movements with looseness of stool.

diuretics: Agents that promote the excretion of urine.

dropsy: A morbid condition characterized by the accumulation of fluid in the serous cavities and connective tissues of the body.

dyspnea: Breathlessness or shortness of breath.

emetics: Agents that cause vomiting.

enemogogues: Agents introduced into the rectum that cause evacuation of the bowel.

enzymes: A substance that promotes a chemical reaction in the body without itself being changed or destroyed. Those that are secreted into the intestine play an essential role in the digestion of food.

erysipelas: A local febrile infection accompanied by diffused inflammation of the skin, causing a deep red colour.

eustachian tube: A channel about 3.6 cm long that connects the middle ear with the nasopharynx. Its functions are to adjust pressure changes in the middle ear and to clear discharges.

exocrine: A body gland that discharges its secretions outwardly, rather than inwardly into the blood.

expectorants: Agents that promote the discharge of mucus and secretions from the chest and lungs.

fibromyalgia: Pain in various muscles and joints of the body, sometimes with "trigger points" (specific areas that are tender to palpation).

flight of ideas: A nearly continuous flow of rapid speech that jumps from topic to topic, usually based on discernible associations or plays on words.

fossa of the helix: The long curved depression in the external ear; also called the scapha.

fourth ventricle: A cavity at the base of the brain that is filled with cerebrospinal fluid.

Functional: 1. A disorder associated with a presumed disturbance of physiological function, as distinct from structure. 2. A psychiatric condition that has a psychological rather than an organic cause. 3. A condition of unknown or uncertain cause.

galvanism: The use of a direct electric current for therapeutic purposes.

gonorrhea: A sexually transmitted disease caused by a specific organism. In the male it causes pain and urethral discharge; in the female it may be asymptomatic, or it may cause a vaginal discharge.

gout: A metabolic disorder that causes pain and swelling of certain joints and surrounding tissues.

gumma: A chronic focal manifestation of tertiary syphilis characterized by the formation of tumours of necrotic tissue that can occur in many different organs.

hallucinosis: A state characterized by the presence of hallucinations without other impairment of consciousness.

helix: The posterior free edge of the external ear.

hematemesis: Blood in the vomitus – that is, originating in the stomach.

hemorrhoids: A condition in which the veins in and around the anus or the lower rectum, are dilated. It is commonly associated with bleeding.

hemoptysis: Blood in the sputum – that is, originating in the lungs or the bronchial tree.

hepatic encephalopathy: A disease of the brain accompanied by disturbances of consciousness, caused by the metabolic changes associated with chronic liver disease.

hepatorenal syndrome: Failure of kidney function due to liver disease, commonly cirrhosis associated with jaundice.

hepatitis: A viral infection that affects the liver.

histological: Concerned with the microscopic anatomical structure of tissues.

homeopathy: A therapeutic system in which diseases are treated by minute amounts of drugs that are capable of producing, in healthy persons, symptoms like those of the disease to be treated.

hyperventilation: A condition in which there is an increased amount of air entering the lungs, from rapid and/or deep breathing. It may be caused by anxiety or fear, is often accompanied by physical symptoms, and superficially may simulate asthma.

hypochondria: Contraction of hypochondriasis. A condition in which there is an unusual preoccupation with bodily functions, and the interpretation of normal internal sensations as indicating an abnormality.

inoculation: The introduction into a healthy individual of a disease agent such as virus, with the intention of producing a mild form of the disease, followed by immunity to that disease.

interstitial keratitis: A chronic infective condition of the cornea of the eye.

inflammatory bowel disease: An uncommon, chronic, relapsing disease of the bowel, of unknown cause, characterized by diarrhea, abdominal pain and blood in the stool. There are two subtypes: Crohn's disease affects mainly the small intestine; ulcerative colitis affects mainly the large intestine.

irritable bowel syndrome: A common, relapsing condition characterized by abdominal pain with diarrhea and/or constipation. Although the cause is not known, psychological factors are thought to be contributory.

jaundice: A medical condition commonly caused by liver failure and characterized by yellow appearance of the skin and the sclera of the eyes. The colour is caused by excess bilirubin in the blood and tissues.

Korsakov's psychosis: A medical condition characterized by loss of memory, and the creation of new memories of events that did not occur. It is a complication of chronic alcoholism.

labyrinthitis: An inflammatory condition of the labyrinth part of the internal ear.

lacrimation: The secretion and discharge of tears.

laxatives: Agents that cause evacuation of the lower bowel.

leprosy: A slowly progressive chronic infectious disease characterized by lesions in the skin, nerves, and other organs of the body.

leucorrhea: In present day medicine, a whitish discharge from the vagina. In earlier times this term may have been used to describe a discharge from any body orifice.

lymphatic system: The small vessels that drain the fluid from the tissues of the body and return it to the blood. The fluid within the vessels is called lymph.

macroscopic: Visible with the naked eye.

magnetic resonance imaging (MRI): A method of visualizing soft tissues of the body (including the brain) by applying an external magnetic field that makes it possible to distinguish between hydrogen ions in different environments.

magnetoencephalograph: An instrument for recording magnetic signals proportional to electroencephalographic waves emanating from electrical activity in the brain.

manic-depression: See bipolar disorder.

mastoid process: A prominence at the lower end of the temporal bone of the skull.

materia medica: An older term for what is now called pharmacology, the branch of medical study that deals with drugs, their sources, and their uses.

melancholia: An ancient term for what is now called depression.

neurosis: A group of mental conditions whose core symptom is anxiety. The condition is distressing to the person, there is no loss of contact with reality, and social norms are not violated.

nosology: The science of the classification of diseases.

numerical medicine: An older term for what is now called epidemiology, the science concerned with the study of the factors influencing the frequency and distribution of disease.

otosclerosis: A disease of the bone surrounding the middle ear that involves the stapes, one of the small bones that transmit sound, and interferes with its function. It generally starts during early adult life, affects the two ears asymmetrically, and is gradually progressive. Microsurgery may be effective; otherwise the treatment is sound augmentation.

Paget's disease: A disease of bone that usually starts in middle age, and is marked by increased bone absorption, and excessive attempts at repair. The affected bones become weak, brittle, and deformed. If the skull is involved, the condition may affect the auditory nerve, resulting in deafness.

palpitations: Subjective sensation of one's own heart beat.

pancreatitis: Acute or chronic inflammation of the pancreas most often caused by alcoholism.

paracentesis: Surgical puncture of a body organ with a needle to remove fluid.

paranoia: A condition in which an individual perceives or interprets others as adopting a hostile attitude towards him or her. This perception is more than is warranted by the particular facts and circumstances. In severe cases, it may reach delusional intensity (paranoid delusion).

paronychia: Infection of the tissues surrounding a finger nail.

peritoneum: The membrane lining the abdominal cavity and the organs that it contains. If this membrane becomes infected or inflamed, peritonitis results.

personality disorder: A group of mental conditions that start in adolescence or early adulthood, and are marked by enduring, inflexible, and maladaptive behavioural traits that are very different from social and cultural expectations.

petechia: Small round purple spot caused by hemorrhage into the skin.

petrous bone: The lower, dense portion of the temporal bone of the skull that contains and protects the delicate structures of the inner ear.

photophobia: Abnormal visual intolerance of light.

pleurisy: Inflammation of the pleura, the membranes that line and envelop both lungs.

pneumonia: Inflammation of one or more lobes of the lungs in which there is a heavy accumulation of fluid in the affected areas.

porphyria: A group of metabolic diseases that affect particularly the skin and the nervous system.

positron emission tomography (PET): The recording of gamma rays emitted from the brain after administration of a natural biochemical substance – such as glucose – into which positron-emitting isotropes have been incorporated.

psychopath: An older term for a condition now known as antisocial personality disorder.

psychopathology: The branch of medicine that deals with the causes and nature of all psychiatric illness.

psychosis: A serious mental disorder marked by loss of contact with reality.

psychosomatic: 1. The study of mind-body relationships. 2. Physical symptoms cause by psychological factors.

purgatives: See cathartics.

pustule: A visible collection of pus in or under the skin.

pyelonephritis: An inflammatory condition of the kidneys, usually due to an infection.

quinchina: A drug extracted from the bark of the cinchona tree; also known as quinquina and cinchona. During the nineteenth century it was used in a wide variety of conditions, and also as a tonic. It is now used mainly as an anti-malarial agent.

racing thoughts: See flights of ideas.

renal papillary necrosis: A disease of the kidneys in which there is death of the tissues in central parts of the organ. It occurs most frequently in people with diabetes mellitus in which the kidneys are secondarily affected.

rheumatism: Any of a group of conditions marked by inflammation or degeneration of connective tissue structures in the body, in particular the bones, muscles, and joints.

sarcoidosis: A chronic and progressive condition characterized by the formation of tumour-like lesions in various organs of the body; also called sarcoid.

scirrhus: In present day medicine, a particular form of cancer of the stomach. In earlier times this term was used to describe a diseased organ or tissue that had a hard or indurated consistency.

schizophrenia: A group of mental disorders in which an individual loses contact with reality (i.e. becomes psychotic), and which are characterized by particular disturbances of thought, mood, and behaviour. Commonly there are also perceptual abnormalities such as hallucinations.

scurvy: A condition characterized by weakness, anemia, and a bleeding tendency, caused by a deficiency of vitamin C in the diet.

smallpox: An acute, contagious, and often fatal disease caused by a virus. It was very common in the eighteenth century, but now has been eliminated by widespread vaccination.

syphilis: A sexually transmitted infective disease caused by an organism called treponema pallidum. Its course falls into three stages: the primary stage affects mainly the genitalia; the secondary stage affects mainly the skin causing widespread skin rashes; in the tertiary stage, which often arrives years after the first two stages, serious diseases of the heart, brain, and other tissues may occur. The formation of one or more "gummata" – tumour-like lesions – in various organs is also typical in the tertiary stage. Syphilis was common in the pre-antibiotic era of medicine.

system: A set or a series of interconnected or interdependent organs in the body that function together in a common purpose: for example, the nervous system, which consists of the brain, spinal cord, and the peripheral and autonomic nerves.

systemic lupus erythematosis: A chronic, relapsing, inflammatory disease that can affect many organs of the body, including particularly the skin, joints, kidneys, and mucus membranes.

tuberculosis: An infectious disease caused by a specific organism; although many organs of the body can be affected, it tends to involve particularly the lungs. It was common in the pre-antibiotic era of medicine, especially in association with overcrowding and poor socio-economic circumstances.

tympanic membrane: The thin partition between the external ear and the tympanic cavity of the middle ear; also called the eardrum.

typhus fever: A group of diseases caused by a bacteria-like organism that is transmitted to humans by certain insects. It causes headaches, skin-rashes, fever, and sometimes inflammation of the brain. It is a rare cause of nerve-type deafness.

vaccination: The introduction of a vaccine into the body for the purpose of inducing immunity to a disease.

vascularization: The process by which an area of the body becomes invaded by blood vessels and cells.

venereal disease: A group of diseases that are transmitted sexually, for example, syphilis and gonorrhea.

venesection: The process of inserting a needle or a knife into a vein for the purpose of withdrawing blood.

vesicatories: An agent that causes blistering of the skin.

Wernicke's encephalopathy: A disease of the brain characterized by confusion, apathy, drowsiness, and other features. It is caused by thiamine (vitamin B1) deficiency, and is commonly associated with alcoholism.

Whipple's disease: A rare disease caused by a specific organism, and characterized by diarrhea, skin pigmentation, anemia, joint symptoms, and the malabsorption of nutrients from the gastrointestinal tract.

Beethoven's Medical History

The following summary of Beethoven's medical history is presented in the format of a medical teaching meeting known as a clinical-pathological conference. At such meetings, a case is presented to a group of physicians by a pathologist who has carried out an autopsy on an individual, and therefore knows the diagnosis (or diagnoses) of the conditions that caused the individual's death. These conferences are used as an exercise in problem solving, because they train clinicians to consider all diagnostic possibilities when reviewing a patient's medical history. At the end of the meeting the pathologist reveals the correct "answers" – the results of the autopsy.

Two such conferences have been held to examine Beethoven as a "case," and the proceedings written up in medical journals.[1] However, the following case history has not been based on the clinical findings presented at those meetings.

MEDICAL HISTORY

Present Illness: The patient was a man of fifty-seven who was deaf and looked older than his years. He had had symptoms of weakness and shortness of breath for several weeks and had recently taken to his bed because of this. He also had had weight loss and swelling of his abdomen and legs.

---

1 Alterman, "Diagnostic Challenge"; Donnenberg, Collins, et al. "The Sound That Failed."

Examination showed clinical evidence of jaundice and ascites. His condition deteriorated and one month later the abdominal fluid was tapped. A large quantity of cloudy fluid was released with short-term symptomatic relief. However the ascites recurred and had to be tapped on three further occasions over the next two months. His condition progressed and was accompanied by anxiety, malaise, and loss of a large amount of weight. Terminally he became delirious, lost consciousness, and died three and a half months after taking to his bed.

Past Health: He had a long history of health problems. His hearing loss began in his late twenties, initially accompanied by extraneous sounds such as humming and buzzing. It was progressive and deafness was nearly complete by age forty-eight.

From age twenty-five he had recurrent episodes of "colic" – indigestion, abdominal pains, frequently accompanied by bloodless diarrhea lasting several days.

He also had recurring episodes of melancholia the first of which occurred at 17 following the death of his mother. There were further episodes at thirty-two (accompanied by suicidal ideation), thirty-nine, forty-two, forty-three, forty-six (with suicidality), forty-seven, forty-eight, fifty-four, and fifty-six. At times, others noted him to be irritable, easily roused to anger, euphoric, overactive, and oversensitive. He was also noted to be suspicious to the point that he felt that his "enemies" were following him.

At various other times during his lifetime he had symptoms such as weakness, exhaustion, insomnia, headaches, pains in his feet and his eyes, "rheumatism," pains in his chest and back, "catarrh," cough, and shakiness. He also experienced recurrent upper respiratory tract infections.

At age fifty-one he had an episode of jaundice that lasted six weeks. It cleared completely and did not recur until his final illness, although episodes of colic and diarrhea appeared to become more frequent thereafter. He had episodes of nosebleeds at fifty-four and fifty-five.

Family Health: His father died at age fifty-two from alcohol related problems. A paternal grandmother also died of alcoholism. His mother died at age forty-one from tuberculosis, as did a younger brother also in his early forties.

Social History: There was disagreement as to whether or not he abused alcohol. He enjoyed wine and fortified wine but was not known to use liquor. He enjoyed parties with friends and this may have been associated with excesses at times, but he was not described as a drunkard. In his final illness his physicians attempted unsuccessfully to ban alcohol but eventually allowed him to take limited quantities of wine with symptomatic relief. Some of his physicians considered that he had overused alcohol, but his friends denied this.

He never married, and although he had transient "affairs" and on occasion may have consorted with prostitutes, he was not known to be sexually promiscuous.

Autopsy Report: The skin showed petechial hemorrhages. The abdominal cavity was filled with a large quantity of a reddish cloudy fluid. The liver was half its normal size, was bluish green in colour, and covered by nodules a few millimeters in diameter. It had a leathery consistency. The gall bladder was filled with gravel like material. The spleen was twice its normal size, compact, and black in colour. The pancreas was also larger than normal and compacted. The stomach and intestines were dilated with air but otherwise normal. Both kidneys were pale red and softened, and there were "calcareous concretions" in each calyx. They were covered with tissue about one inch thick and this contained a dark cloudy fluid. The thoracic cavity and heart appeared normal. Histological sections were not available.

Toxicological analysis of a sample of hair many years after his death showed markedly elevated levels of lead, but an absence of mercury, arsenic, and narcotics.

Criteria for Alcohol Dependence and Abuse[1]

CRITERIA FOR ALCOHOL DEPENDENCE

A maladaptive pattern of alcohol use, leading to clinically significant impairment or distress, as manifested by three (or more) of the following, occurring any time in the same twelve month period.

1   tolerance, as defined by either of the following:
    a   a need for markedly increased amounts of alcohol to achieve intoxication or the desired effect.
    b   markedly diminished effect with continued use of the same amount of alcohol.
2   withdrawal, as manifested by either of the following:
    a   the characteristic withdrawal syndrome for alcohol.
    b   the same (or a closely related) substance is taken to relieve or avoid the withdrawal symptoms.
3   alcohol is often taken in larger amounts or over a longer period than was intended.

---

1   American Psychiatric Association: *Diagnostic and Statistical Manual of Mental Disorders*, 181–3. Minor modifications from the original text have been made. In particular, the word "substance" in the original has been changed to "alcohol," because in this context, we are concerned only with alcohol misuse, not the misuse of other habit-forming substances.

4   there is a persistent desire or unsuccessful efforts to cut down or control
    alcohol use.
5   a great deal of time is spent in activities necessary to obtain alcohol, or
    recover from its effects.
6   important social, occupational, or recreational activities are given up or
    reduced because of alcohol use.
7   alcohol use is continued despite knowledge of having a persistent or recur-
    rent physical or psychological problem that is likely to have been caused or
    exacerbated by its use.

CRITERIA FOR ALCOHOL ABUSE

A   A maladaptive pattern of alcohol use leading to clinically significant impair-
    ment or distress, as manifested by one (or more) of the following, occurring
    within a twelve-month period:

1   recurrent alcohol use resulting in failure to fulfill major role obligations at
    work, school, or home (e.g., repeated absences or poor work performance
    related to alcohol use; alcohol-related absences, suspensions, or expul-
    sions from school; neglect of children or household).
2   recurrent alcohol use in situations in which it is physically hazardous (e.g.,
    driving an automobile or operating a machine when impaired).
3   recurrent alcohol related legal problems (e.g., arrest or alcohol related dis-
    orderly conduct)
4   continued alcohol use despite having persistent or recurrent social or
    interpersonal problems caused or exacerbated by its use (e.g., argument
    with a spouse about consequences of intoxication, physical fights)

B   The symptoms have never met the criteria for alcohol dependence.

Dr Andreas Wawruch's Medical Report[1]

Ludwig van Beethoven declared that from earliest youth he had possessed a rugged, permanently good constitution, hardened by many privations, which even the most strenuous toil at his favourite occupation and continual profound study had been unable in the slightest degree to impair. The lonely nocturnal quiet always had shown itself most friendly to his glowing imagination. Hence he usually wrote after midnight until about three o'clock. A short sleep of from four to five hours was all he needed to refresh him. His breakfast eaten, he sat down at his writing desk again until two o'clock in the afternoon.

When he entered his thirtieth year, however, he began to suffer from haemorrhoidal complaints and an annoying roaring and buzzing in both ears. Soon his hearing began to fail, and, for all he often would enjoy untroubled intervals lasting for months at a time, his disability finally ended in complete deafness. All the resources of the physician's art were useless. At about the same time Beethoven noticed that his digestion began to suffer; loss of appetite was followed by indigestion, an annoying belching, an alternate obstinate constipation, and frequent diarrhea.

At no time accustomed to taking medical advice seriously, he began to develop a liking for spirituous beverages, in order to stimulate his decreasing appetite and to aid his stomachic weakness by excessive use of strong punch and iced drinks

---

1 This report is taken from Nettl, *The Beethoven Encyclopedia*, 40–3.

and long, tiring excursions on foot. It was this very alteration of his mode of life which, some seven years earlier, had led him to the brink of the grave. He contracted a severe inflammation of the intestines, which though it yielded to treatment, later on often gave rise to intestinal pains and aching colics and which, in part, must have favoured the eventual development of his mortal illness.

In the late fall of the year just passed (1826) Beethoven felt an irresistible urge, in view of the uncertain state of his health, to go to the country to recuperate. Since owing to his incurable deafness he sedulously avoided society, he was thrown entirely upon his own resources under the most unfavourable circumstances for days and even weeks at a time. Often with rare endurance, he worked at his compositions on a wooded hillside and his work done, still aglow with reflection, he would not infrequently run about for hours in the most inhospitable surroundings, defying every change of temperature, and often during the heaviest snowfalls. His feet, always from time to time edematous, would begin to swell and since (as he insisted) he had to do without every comfort of life, every solacing refreshment, his illness soon got the upper hand of him.

Intimidated by the sad prospect, in the gloomy future, of finding himself helpless in the country should he fall sick, he longed to be back in Vienna, and, as he himself jovially said, used the devil's own most wretched conveyance, a milk-wagon, to carry him home.

December was raw, wet, cold, and frosty. Beethoven's clothing was anything but suited to the unkind season of the year, and yet he was driven on and away by an inner restlessness, a sinister presentiment of misfortune. He was obliged to stop overnight in a village inn, when in addition to the shelter afforded by its wretched roof he found only an unheated room without winter windows. Toward midnight he was seized with his first convulsive chills and fever, accompanied by violent thirst and pains in the side. When the fever heat began to break, he drank a couple of quarts of ice-cold water, and, in his helpless state, yearned for the first ray of dawn. Weak and ill, he had himself loaded on the open van and, finally, arrived in Vienna enervated and exhausted.

I was not sent for until the third day. I found Beethoven with grave symptoms of inflammation of the lungs; his face glowed, he spit blood, when he breathed he threatened to choke, and the shooting pain in his side only allowed him to lie in a tormenting posture flat on his back. A strict anti-inflammatory mode of treatment soon brought the desired amelioration; nature conquered and a happy crisis freed him of the seemingly imminent danger of death, so that on the fifth day he was able to sit up and relate to me with deep emotion the story of the adversities he had suffered. On the seventh day he felt so passably well that he could rise, move about, read and write. Yet on the eighth day I was not a little alarmed. On my morning visit I found him quite upset; his entire body jaundiced; while a terrible fit of vomiting and diarrhea during the preceding night had threatened to kill him. Violent anger, profound suffering because of ingratitude, and an undeserved insult had motivated the tremendous explosion. Shaking and trembling, he writhed with the pain which raged in his liver and intestines; and his feet, hitherto only moderately puffed up, were now greatly swollen.

From this time on his dropsy developed; his secretions decreased in quantity, his liver gave convincing evidence of the presence of hard knots, his jaundice grew worse. The affectionate remonstrance of his friends soon appeased the threatening excitement and Beethoven, easily conciliated, soon forgot every insult offered him. His illness, however, progressed with giant strides. Already, during the third week, nocturnal choking attacks set in, the tremendous volume of the water accumulated called for immediate relief; and I found myself compelled to advocate the abdominal puncture in order to preclude the danger of sudden bursting. After a few moments of serious reflection Beethoven agreed to submit to the operation, the more so since Ritter von Staudenheim, who had been called in as consulting physician, urgently recommended it as being imperatively necessary. The premier surgeon of the General Hospital, the Mag. Chir. Hr. Seibert, made the puncture with his habitual skill, so that Beethoven when he saw the stream of water cried out happily that the operation made him think of Moses, who struck the rock with his staff and made the water gush forth. The relief was almost immediate. The liquid amounted to twenty-five pounds in weight, yet the afterflow must have been five times that.

Carelessness in undoing the bandage of the wound at night, probably in order quickly to remove all the water which had gathered, well nigh put an end to all rejoicing anent (sic) the improvement in Beethoven's condition. A violent erysipelatic inflammation set in and showed incipient signs of gangrene, but the greatest care exercised in keeping the inflamed surfaced dry soon checked the evil. Fortunately the three succeeding operations were carried out without the slightest difficulty.

Beethoven knew but too well that the tappings were only palliatives and hence resigned himself to a further accumulation of water, the more so since the cold, rainy winter season favoured the return of his dropsy, and could not help but strengthen the original cause of his illness, which had its existence in his chronic liver trouble as well as in organic deficiencies of the abdominal intestines.

It is a curious fact that Beethoven, even after operations successfully performed, could not stand taking any medicine, if we except gentle laxatives. His appetite diminished from day to day, and his strength could not help but decrease noticeably in consequence of the repeated large loss of vital juices. Dr. Malfatti, who henceforth aided me with his advice, a friend of Beethoven's for many years and aware of the latter's inclination for spirituous beverages, therefore hit upon the idea of recommending iced punch. I must admit that his recipe worked admirably, for a few days at any rate. Beethoven felt so greatly refreshed by the iced spirits of wine that he slept through the whole of the first night, and began to sweat tremendously. He grew lively; often all sorts of witty ideas occurred to him; and he even dreamt of being able to complete the oratorio *Saul and David* which he had commenced.

Yet, as was to have been foreseen, his joy was of short duration. He began to abuse his prescription, and partook freely of the punch. Soon the alcoholic beverage called forth a powerful rush of blood to the head; he grew soporose and there was a rattle when he breathed like that of a person deeply intoxicated; he wandered in his talk and to this, at various times, was added in inflammatory pain in the neck with consequent hoarseness and even total speechlessness. He grew more violent and now, since colic and diarrhea had resulted from the chilling of the intestines, it was high time to deprive him of this valuable stimulant.

It was under such conditions, together with a rapidly increasing loss of flesh and a noticeable falling off of his vital powers that January, February, and March went by. Beethoven in gloomy hours of presentiment foretold his approaching dissolution after his fourth tapping, nor was he mistaken. No consolation was able longer to revive him; and when I promised him that with the approaching spring weather his sufferings would decrease, he answered with a smile: "My day's work is done; if a physician still can be of use in my case" (and then he lapsed into English) "his name shall be called wonderful." This saddening reference to Handel's *Messiah* so profoundly moved me that in my inmost soul and with the deepest emotion I was obliged to confirm the truth of what he had said.

And now the ill-fated day drew ever nearer. My noble and often burdensome professional duty as a physician bade me call my suffering friend's attention to the momentous day, so that he might comply with his civic and religious duties. With the most delicate consideration I set down the admonitory lines on a sheet of paper (for it was thus that we always had made ourselves mutually understood). Beethoven, slowly, meditatively and with incomparable self-control read what I had written, his face like that of one transfigured. Next he gave me his hand in a hearty, serious manner and said: "Have them send for his reverence the pastor." Then he grew quiet and reflective, and nodded me his: "I shall soon see you again," in friendly wise. Soon after Beethoven attended to his devotions with the pious resignation which looks forward with confidence to eternity.

When a few hours had passed, he lost consciousness, began to grow comatose, and breathed with a rattle. The following morning all symptoms pointed to the approaching end. The 26th of March was stormy, and clouded. Toward six in the afternoon came a flurry of snow, with thunder and lightning – Beethoven died. Would not a Roman augur, in view of the accidental commotion of the elements, have taken his apotheosis for granted?

NOTES

CHAPTER ONE

1 Albrecht, *Letters to Beethoven and Other Correspondence*, 1: 22.
2 Wegeler and Ries, *Beethoven Remembered*, 68; Lockwood, *Beethoven*, 210–12, questions the accuracy of Ries's description of this event.
3 Ferdinand II was Holy Roman Emperor from 1619 to 1637. See DeNora, *Beethoven and the Construction of Genius*, 39–40.
4 Rice, "Vienna under Joseph II and Leopold II."
5 Marek, *Beethoven*, 23–36.
6 Mellers, *Beethoven and the Voice of God*, 5.
7 Thayer, *Thayer's Life of Beethoven*, 33.
8 Will and Ariel Durant, *Rousseau and Revolution*, 531–628.
9 Shackleton, "Enlightenment."
10 Kinderman, *Beethoven*, 7.
11 Krieger, *Kings and Philosophers*, 230.
12 Kinderman, *Beethoven*, 7.
13 Libby, "Italy."
14 Rousseau, "Léttre sur la musique française," 62–80.
15 Davies, Norman, *Europe*, 604–5.
16 Krieger, *Kings and Philosophers*, 160; As a group, they could be described more as social reformers than philosophers; Hume was the only fully fledged philosopher amongst them.

17 Rousseau, "Léttre sur la musique française," 62–80; Didier, *La musique des lumières.*

18 Mongrédien, "Paris."

19 Shackleton, "Enlightenment," 260.

20 Will and Ariel Durant, *The Age of Voltaire*, 635.

21 Furbank, *Diderot*, 242–58.

22 The States-General was a convocation that represented the three levels of French society: the nobility, the church, and the people)

23 Anderson, *Letters* [of Beethoven], 1: 96.

24 Herriot, *La vie de Beethoven*, 120–8.

25 Thayer, *Thayer's Life of Beethoven*, 578.

26 Spiel, *The Congress of Vienna*, 242–3.

27 Davies, *Europe*, 762.

28 Braudel, *The Structures of Everyday Life*, 479–558.

29 The term laissez-faire expresses the principle that governments should not interfere with the actions of individuals in industrial affairs and in trade.

30 W. and A. Durant, *The Age of Voltaire*, 274–7.

31 Braudel, *Structures of Everyday Life*, 424–5.

32 Pinel, *Nosographie philosophique*, 1: 40–4.

33 Baillie, *The Morbid Anatomy*, 15.

34 "Numerical medicine" – the use of careful observation and the counting of frequencies in a clinical setting – is the forerunner of the modern sciences of epidemiology and medical statistics. See Sournia, *Illustrated History of Medicine*, 340–2.

35 Pfeiffer, *Art and Practice of Western Medicine*, 46.

36 Pinel, *Nosographie philosophique*, 1: 40–4.

37 Thomson, *New Guide To Health*, 105.

38 A complete translation of this letter is given in chapter 3.

39 Williams, *Treatise on the Ear*, 208–55.

40 Sournia, *Illustrated History of Medicine*, 340–2.

41 Pinel, *Nosographie philosophique*, 1: lxxxiii–lxxxv.

42 Chapman, *Elements of Therapeutics and Materia Medica.*

43 Fischer-Homberger, "E. Germany and Austria."

44 Jenner, *An Inquiry into the Causes and Effects of Cow Pox.*

45 Maehle, "Conflicting Attitudes towards Inoculation," 198–222.

46 Withering, *An Account of the Foxglove.*

47 Sournia, *Illustrated History of Medicine*, 316.

48 Pfeiffer, *Art and Practice of Western Medicine*, 198.

49 Ibid., 10.

50 Sournia, *Illustrated History of Medicine*, 339–40.

51 Beaumont, *Physiology of Digestion*; Mai, "Beaumont's Contribution to Gastric Psychophysiology."

52 Jordanova, "Reflections on Medical Reform."

53 Lindemann, *Health and Healing in Eighteenth-Century Germany*, 263–4.

54 Krizek, "History of Balneotherapy."

55 Coley, "Physicians, Chemists and the Analysis of Mineral Waters."

56 Scheminsky, "Austria."

57 Tourtelle, *Élémens d'hygiène*.

58 Ibid.; an example of an exaggerated claim is: "Inactivity is the fatal source from which come most of the calamities that afflict the human species." 2: 381.

59 Broman, *Transformation of German Academic Medicine*, 128–58.

60 Frank, *System einer vollständigen medizenischen Polizey*; Broman, *Transformation of German Academic Medicine*, 114–19.

61 Anderson, Beethoven *Letters*, 3: 1371.

62 Thayer, *Thayer's Life of Beethoven*, 946.

63 Knight, *Beethoven and the Age of Revolution*, 36–46.

64 Marx, "Beethoven, l'homme politique."

65 Schindler, *Beethoven As I Knew Him*, 112–20 and 243–8.

66 Knight, *Beethoven and the Age of Revolution*, 148.

67 Ibid., 36–46.

68 Nettl, *The Beethoven Encyclopedia*, 195–8.

69 Thayer, *Thayer's Life of Beethoven*, 800

70 Knight, *Beethoven and the Age of Revolution*, 111–16; the Conversation Books were the books used by Beethoven's friends to communicate with him in writing after he became too deaf to engage in verbal dialogue.

71 Ibid., 139–45.

72 Prod'homme, *Cahiers de conversation*, 400–17 (my translation).

73 Knight, *Beethoven and the Age of Revolution*, 111–16.

74 Lockwood, *Beethoven: The Music and the Life*, 152.

75 Ibid., 400–17.

76 Buch, *Beethoven's Ninth*, 4–5.

CHAPTER TWO

1 Anderson, Beethoven *Letters*, 1: 66-8.
2 These three periods cover Beethoven's years in Vienna, 1792–1827, with 1802, the year of the Heilegenstadt Testament, as the transition point between the first and second periods, and 1812, the year of his letters to the "Immortal Beloved," as the transition between the second and third periods. A number of scholars, however, disagree with 1812 as the start of the third period. The years 1812–16 were a fallow period during which Beethoven wrote relatively little music. The composition that marked the start of his third period was Sonata no. 28, op. 101, written in 1816 and published early in 1817. In some respects, the death of his brother Carl in 1815 was a more seminal emotional event for him than the fracture of his relationship with the "Immortal Beloved" in 1812, not so much because of his brother's death per se but because of the ensuing legal battle with his sister-in-law over the custody of his nephew Karl. This battle was to pre-occupy Beethoven's mind and attention for four years, and his relationship with Karl was to be the predominant one for the rest of his life. For these reasons, the four years from 1812 to 1816 may best be regarded as a period of transition between the second and third periods, with composition of op. 101 marking the formal beginning of the third period. For further discussion on this point, see Lockwood, *Beethoven*; Kerman and Tyson, *The New Grove Beethoven*, 89–91.
3 Kinderman, *Beethoven*, 1–14.
4 Thayer, *Thayer's Life of Beethoven*, 41
5 Closson, *L'élément flamand dans Beethoven*, chap. 2.
6 Thayer, *Thayer's Life of Beethoven*, 12.
7 Ibid., 42.
8 Wegeler and Ries, *Beethoven Remembered*, 13.
9 Fischer, in Sonneck, *Beethoven*, 3–10.
10 Wegeler and Ries, *Beethoven Remembered*, 13.
11 Thayer, *Thayer's Life of Beethoven*, 51.
12 Ibid., 59; Fischer, in Sonneck, *Beethoven*, 7.
13 Thayer, *Thayer's Life of Beethoven*, 68.
14 Ibid., 65.
15 Neefe, in Sonneck, *Beethoven*, 10.
16 Wegeler and Ries, *Beethoven Remembered*, 13.

17 Marek, *Beethoven*, 65.

18 Wegeler and Ries, *Beethoven Remembered*, 14.

19 Wegeler, in Albrecht, *Letters to Beethoven and Other Correspondence*, 3: 120–6.

20 Wegeler describes an evening in 1810 when Bettina Brentano wrote down everything Beethoven had told him: "This morning I read it to him," and he said: "Did I really say that? Well then, I had a raptus again." (Wegeler and Ries, *Beethoven Remembered*, 39).

21 Schindler, *Beethoven As I Knew Him*, 47.

22 The Zehrgarten was a tavern that Beethoven and his friends frequented. When he left Bonn for Vienna in 1792, fourteen of them presented him with a "Stammbuch" (autograph book) in which each of them had inscribed a personal message. Beethoven treasured this book until his death. See Breuning, in Albrecht, *Letters to Beethoven and Other Correspondence*, 1: 14.

23 Anderson, Beethoven *Letters*, 1: 9–11.

24 Ibid., 1: 13–15.

25 Ibid., 1: 57–62 and 66–8.

26 Ibid., 1: 113–14.

27 Von Breuning, *Memories of Beethoven*.

28 Anderson, Beethoven *Letters*, 1: 113–14; Karl Amenda (1771–1836) was the living friend, Lorenz the friend who had died.

29 Nothing is known of Beethoven's meeting with the emperor, if indeed it took place, and his meeting with Mozart, while probable, has also not been confirmed. There is a possibly apocryphal story that after hearing Beethoven play, Mozart wrote, "Keep your eyes on him; some day he will give the world something to talk about." See Küster, *Mozart*, 189; Mozart, in Sonneck, *Beethoven*, 11.

30 Anderson, Beethoven *Letters*, 1: 3–4.

31 Ibid.; Marek, *Beethoven: Biography of a Genius*, 76.

32 Wegeler and Ries, *Beethoven Remembered*, 65.

33 Ibid., 109.

34 Anderson, Beethoven *Letters*, 1: 57–62.

35 Thayer, *Thayer's Life of Beethoven*, 122.

36 Ibid., 128.

37 The Zehrgarten Stammbuch for Beethoven, in Albrecht, *Letters to Beethoven and Other Correspondence*, 1: 15–29.

38 Webster, "The Falling-out between Haydn and Beethoven," 3–45.

39 Wegeler and Ries, *Beethoven Remembered*, 75.

40 Ibid., 24.

41 Ibid., 34; Anderson, Beethoven *Letters*, 1: 9–11.

42 Wegeler and Ries, *Beethoven Remembered*, 24.

43 Ibid., 82; as noted above, Ries' father had helped the Beethoven family at the time of Beethoven's mother's death in 1787.

44 The "Eroica" symphony was published in 1804 as op. 55; Beethoven's feeling of betrayal when Napoleon crowned himself emperor is described in chapter 1.

45 Anderson, Beethoven *Letters*, 1: 57–62.

46 Thayer, *Thayer's Life of Beethoven*, 232.

47 Anderson, Beethoven *Letters*, 1: 66–8.

48 Prod'homme, *Cahiers de conversation*, 228 (my translation).

49 Anderson, Beethoven *Letters*, 1: 57–62.

50 Wegeler and Ries, *Beethoven Remembered*, 86.

51 Von Breuning, *Memories of Beethoven*, 37.

52 Anderson, Beethoven *Letters*, 1: 63–5.

53 N. Zmeskall, in Nettl, *The Beethoven Encyclopedia*, 313.

54 Thayer, *Thayer's Life of Beethoven*, xiv.

55 With minor variations, this extract is taken from a translation by Marek, *Beethoven*, 325–7.

56 Kinderman, *Beethoven*, 1–14; Tovey, *Beethoven*, 5–52.

57 Thayer, *Thayer's Life of Beethoven*, 670.

58 Cooper, *Beethoven*, 257.

59 Von Breuning, *Memories of Beethoven*, 44.

60 Barry Cooper's edition is the first English translation of this work. In his introduction Cooper notes that although there are major omissions in this biography, it paints an accurate portrait of Beethoven.

61 Schlosser, *Beethoven*, 87–8.

62 Wegeler and Ries, *Beethoven Remembered*, 42.

63 Ibid., 104.

64 Schindler, *Beethoven As I Knew Him*, 246 and 231.

65 Ibid., 56.

66 Ibid., 121.

67 Josephine Deym, in Albrecht, *Letters to Beethoven and Other Correspondence*, 1: 160–4.

68   Anderson, Beethoven *Letters*, 1: 130–2.

69   Ibid., 1: 134.

70   Ibid., 1: 134–5.

71   Ibid., 1: 135–6.

72   Josephine Deym, in Albrecht, *Letters to Beethoven and Other Correspondence*, 1: 160.

73   Ibid., 1: 162.

74   Rolland, *Le chant de la resurrection*, 251–5.

75   Anderson, Beethoven *Letters*, 1: 167, 175–6, 177–9.

76   Ibid., 1: 161.

77   Ibid., 1: 162–3 and 163–5.

78   Jeanclaude, *Un amour de Beethoven*.

79   Anderson, Beethoven *Letters*, 1: 223–4.

80   Anna-Marie Erdödy, in Albrecht, *Letters to Beethoven and Other Correspondence*, 2: 75–6.

81   Anderson, Beethoven *Letters*, 2: 579.

82   Ibid., 2: 527–8.

83   Ibid., 2: 683–4.

84   Ibid., 1: 272–4.

85   Ibid., 1: 270–1.

86   Ibid., 1: 268–9.

87   Thayer, *Thayer's Life of Beethoven*, 686.

88   Anderson has pointed out that the German phrase, *Unsterbliche Geliebte*, by which Beethoven addressed the woman in one of the letters, is more correctly translated as "Eternally Beloved"; Anderson, Beethoven *Letters*, 1, note on p. 376.

89   Anderson, Beethoven *Letters,*1: 373–6.

90   Marek, *Beethoven*, 295–311.

91   Rolland, *Le chant de la resurrection*, 1475–95.

92   Schindler, *Beethoven As I Knew Him*, 105.

93   Solomon, *Beethoven*, 158–89.

94   Marek, *Beethoven*, 305–7.

95   Rolland, *Le chant de la resurrection*, 1488.

96   Anderson, Beethoven *Letters*, 2: 557–8.

97   Antonie Brentano, in Albrecht, *Letters to Beethoven and Other Correspondence*, 2: 156–7.

98   Lund, "Beethoven."

99 Rolland, *Le chant de la reurrection*, 821–4.

100 Solomon, *Beethoven*, 183 footnote.

101 Thayer, *Thayer's Life of Beethoven*, 549. This prayer is referred to in the Tagebuch of the Fischoff manuscript.

102 Bettina Brentano, in Sonneck, *Beethoven*, 79–88.

103 W. Goethe, in Sonneck, *Beethoven*, 88.

104 Thayer, *Thayer's Life of Beethoven*, 537.

105 Rolland, *Le chant de la resurrection*, 273–412.

106 Anderson, Beethoven *Letters*, 1: 22–3.

107 Knight, *Beethoven and the Age of Revolution*, 70.

108 Thayer, *Thayer's Life of Beethoven*, 542.

109 Anderson, Beethoven *Letters*, 1: 142–3.

110 Ibid., 1: 185–6 and 193–4.

111 Ibid., 1: 274–5.

112 Ibid., 1: 270–1.

113 Ibid., 1: 430–1.

114 Thayer, *Thayer's Life of Beethoven*, 550–1.

115 Ibid., 456.

116 1 ducat = 4.25 Austrian florins = $US25.00 (1969 value, which is equivalent to $130.00 at 2004 values). See Marek, *Beethoven*, xviii; Thayer, *Thayer's Life of Beethoven*, 457–8.

117 Nettl, *Beethoven Encyclopedia*, 202.

118 Wegeler and Ries, *Beethoven Remembered*, 35.

119 Anderson, Beethoven *Letters*, 1: 422–3; Thayer, *Thayer's Life of Beethoven*, 520.

120 Thayer, *Thayer's Life of Beethoven*, 785–95.

121 H.A. Probst, in Albrecht, *Letters to Beethoven and Other Correspondence*, 3: 53.

122 See Thayer, *Thayer's Life of Beethoven*, 1061–76. A review of Beethoven's estate reveals that his most valuable asset was his bank shares (7,441 florins), and that he also left 1215 florins in cash. His chattels were sold by auction for but 1,229 florins; his total assets were 9,885 florins. The total would be equivalent to about $US315,000 at 2004 values. See also Marek, *Beethoven*, xviii.

123 Thayer, *Thayer's Life of Beethoven*, 1109–10.

124 Anderson, Beethoven *Letters*, 1: 252.

125 Ibid., 2: 750–2.

126 Ibid., 2: 748-9.

127 Thayer, *Thayer's Life of Beethoven*, 551; Wegeler and Ries, *Beethoven Remembered*, 87-8.

128 Quoted in Marek, *Beethoven*, 492-4.

129 Anderson, Beethoven *Letters*, 2: 562-3.

130 Thayer, *Thayer's Life of Beethoven*, 677.

131 Anderson, Beethoven *Letters*, 2: 789.

132 Ibid., 2: 792-3.

133 Schindler, *Beethoven As I Knew Him*, 218.

134 Thayer, *Thayer's Life of Beethoven*, 752.

135 Anderson, Beethoven *Letters*, 2: 577-8.

136 Ibid., 2: 612.

137 Ibid., 2: 584-5.

138 Ibid., 2: 668-9.

139 Ibid., 2: 683-4.

140 Ibid., 2: 691.

141 Ibid., 2: 685-6.

142 Ibid., 2: 701.

143 Ibid., 2: 767-71.

144 Ibid., 3: 1209-12.

145 Sterba and Sterba, *Beethoven and His Nephew*, chap. 2.

146 Ibid., 10.

147 Thayer, *Thayer's Life of Beethoven*, 482-3 and 820-1.

148 Ibid., 670-2.

149 Prod'homme, *Cahiers de conversation*, 100.

150 Anderson, Beethoven *Letters*, 2: 813-15, 846-7, 2: 920-1, 958-9, 978-9; 3: 1014.

151 Von Breuning, *Memories of Beethoven*, 102.

152 Schmidt-Görg, *Ludwig Van Beethoven*, 14-15.

153 Anderson, Beethoven *Letters*, 2: 920-1.

154 Thayer, *Thayer's Life of Beethoven*, 777-8.

155 Schindler, *Beethoven As I Knew Him*, 201.

156 Anderson, Beethoven *Letters*, 3: 1036-7 and 1037-8; Papageno is a character from Mozart's opera *The Magic Flute* whose mouth was padlocked for telling lies.

157 Schindler, *Beethoven As I Knew Him*.

158 Prod'homme, *Cahiers de conversation*, 12-23; Marek, *Beethoven*, 484-6.

159 Anderson, Beethoven *Letters*, 2: 956–7 and 958–9.

160 Schindler, *Beethoven As I Knew Him*, 284–90.

161 Mellers, *Beethoven and the Voice of God*, 291.

162 BIS CD – 406/407.

163 Schindler, *Beethoven As I Knew Him*, 280; The political message conveyed in these two remarkable compositions is discussed in chapter 1.

164 Anderson, Beethoven *Letters*, 3: 1026–7.

165 Ibid., 3: 1037–8.

166 Ibid., 3: 1039–40.

167 Ibid., 3: 1058–9 and 1071.

168 Ibid., 3: 1104–6.

169 Ibid., 3: 1086–7.

170 Ibid., 3: 1205–6.

171 Prod'homme, *Cahiers de conversation*, 295.

172 Ibid., 299.

173 Ibid., 317.

174 Ibid., 333–5.

175 Thayer, *Thayer's Life of Beethoven*, 882.

176 Knight, *Beethoven and the Age of Revolution*, 132.

177 Anderson, Beethoven *Letters*, 3: 1201–2 and 1254–6.

178 Ibid., 3: 1226–7.

179 Theodore Molt brought Beethoven's canon back to Quebec. It is now held by the McGill University Library. Canadian composer Alexander Brott used this canon as a basis for his *Paraphrase in Polyphony* (1967), a Centennial Commission. Molt went on to become a well-known music teacher and organist at the Quebec Basilica and was the first organist to participate in the St Jean Baptiste Day Celebrations in Quebec. See *Beethoven and Quebec*, Lawrence Lande Foundations for Canadian Historical Research Publications 2 (Montreal: Redpath Library, McGill University, 1966).

180 Thayer, *Thayer's Life of Beethoven*, 967.

181 Ibid., 1012–13.

182 Marek, *Beethoven*, 522.

183 Ibid., 523.

184 Prod'homme, *Cahiers de conversation*, 210.

185 Thayer, *Thayer's Life of Beethoven*, 1007.

186 Wawruch wrote a narrative report describing Beethoven's case history and published it six weeks after Beethoven's death. Wawruch likely ob-

tained details of the return journey to Vienna from Karl and Beethoven. All Wawruch's comments described in this chapter, with the exception of those taken directly from the Conversation Books, are from this report. The complete text of the report is given in Appendix 4. See also Nettl, *Beethoven Encyclopedia*, 40–3.

187 Thayer, *Thayer's Life of Beethoven*, 1017 footnote.

188 Prod'homme, *Cahiers de conversation*, 437.

189 Marek, *Beethoven*, 619.

190 Anderson, Beethoven *Letters*, 3: 1320–1.

191 Ibid., 3: 1321–3.

192 Von Breuning, *Memories of Beethoven*, 87.

193 Thayer, *Thayer's Life of Beethoven*, 1023.

194 The Conversation Books report the following questions and comments by Wawruch after the operation: "Do you feel better?" "Was it painful?" "Let me know if you don't feel well?" "God save you" [English in original], "Lie quietly on your side" "Five and one half measures were removed" "I hope that you sleep better tonight" "You behaved very chivalrously." Prod'homme, *Cahiers de conversation*, 442.

195 Anderson, Beethoven *Letters*, 3: 1332–3.

196 Ibid., 3: 1333–4.

197 Ibid., 3: 1339.

198 Ibid., 3: 1343.

199 Prod'homme, *Cahiers de conversation*, 451–71.

200 Nettl, *Beethoven Encyclopedia*, 18.

201 Von Breuning, *Memories of Beethoven*, 44.

202 Ibid., 92.

203 In the early nineteenth century, the need for aseptic technique before surgery was not known; hence wound sepsis after surgery was common.

204 Von Breuning, *Memories of Beethoven*, 93–5.

205 Thayer, *Thayer's Life of Beethoven*, 1028–9.

206 Ibid., 1030.

207 Schindler, *Beethoven As I Knew Him*, 320.

208 Ibid., 457.

209 Schindler, in Sonneck, *Beethoven*, 212–14.

210 Thayer, *Thayer's Life of Beethoven*, 1031.

211 Prod'homme, *Cahiers de conversation*, 456.

212 Anderson, Beethoven *Letters*, 3: 1334.

213 Ibid., 3: 1346; Beethoven substituted the word "natural" for "legitimate" in the document.

214 Thayer, *Thayer's Life of Beethoven*, 1049; " with the greatest readiness … have the priest called."

215 Schindler, *Beethoven As I Knew Him*, 324.

216 Thayer, *Thayer's Life of Beethoven*, 1050.

217 Von Breuning, *Memories of Beethoven*, 102–4.

218 Schindler, *Beethoven As I Knew Him*, 324.

219 Ibid., 325.

220 Von Breuning, *Memories of Beethoven*, 104.

221 Thayer, *Thayer's Life of Beethoven*, 1072–6.

222 Albrecht, *Letters to Beethoven and Other Correspondence*, 3: 1072–6.

223 Von Breuning, *Memories of Beethoven*, 108.

224 Gerhard von Breuning poignantly describes his thoughts and feelings as he examined Beethoven's skull in 1863, thirty-six years after his death, at the time of the first exhumation; von Breuning, *Memories of Beethoven*, 118.

CHAPTER THREE

1 Anderson, Beethoven *Letters*, 1: 268–9, written in the spring of 1810.

2 Shedlock, *Beethoven's Letters*.

3 Anderson, Beethoven *Letters*. Anderson's edition is the most recent English edition of Beethoven's letters. There is, however, a more recent and comprehensive compilation of Beethoven letters in the original German, edited by Sieghard Brandenburg, *Beethoven: Briefwechsel Gesamtausgabe*; this edition was not used for the present analysis.

4 Anderson, Beethoven *Letters*, xviii–xxi; Marek, *Beethoven*, 42.

5 Anderson, Beethoven *Letters*, 1: 480 and 482–3.

6 Ibid., 1: 63–5 and 222.

7 Ibid., 2: 519–20.

8 Ibid., 1: 169–70, 316, and 480. Beethoven may have incorrectly dated the first of these letters as 13 June (see Anderson 1: 171n4); the correct date is likely 22 July 1807, and this correction is confirmed by the fact that in a letter of 26 July 1807 (Anderson, 1: 174), he complains of an "illness which affected my head."

9 Ibid., 1: 300. In this letter he states "On account of my foot I cannot walk so far." No further details are provided.

10 Ibid., 1: 342 – "My feet are better." Again, no details are provided.

11 Ibid., 2: 716 refers to "frightful attack of rheumatism."

12 Ibid., 2: 915–16.

13 Ibid., 3: 1278.

14 Ibid., 1: 186–8.

15 Ibid., 2: 944–5.

16 Johann Schmidt, quoted in Thayer, *Ludwig van Beethovens Leben*, 3: 33; a translation of this letter made by Anne Weiser is on p. 167. See also Prod'homme, *Cahiers de conversation de Beethoven*, 379.

17 Anderson, Beethoven *Letters*, 1: 3–4.

18 Ibid., 1: 395.

19 Albrecht, *Letters to Beethoven and Other Correspondence.*

20 Stephan Breuning, in Albrecht, *Letters to Beethoven and Other Correspondence*, 1: 148.

21 Schindler, *Beethoven As I Knew Him*, 62–3.

22 Ibid., 238–9.

23 Karl Beethoven, in Albrecht, *Letters to Beethoven and Other Correspondence*, 3: 107.

24 T. Haslinger, in Albrecht, *Letters to Beethoven and Other Correspondence*, 3: 419.

25 Ibid., 3: 200–12.

26 Carl Czerny, in Sonneck, *Beethoven*, 30.

27 I. Ignaz von Seyfried, in Sonneck, *Beethoven*, 38–9.

28 Wegeler and Ries, *Beethoven Remembered*, 109.

29 F. Rochlitz, in Sonneck, *Beethoven*, 121.

30 L. Schlosser, in Sonneck, *Beethoven*, 144.

31 *Ludwig Van Beethovens Konversatione Hefte.*

32 Prod'homme, *Cahiers de conversation*: all quotations from this work are my translations.

33 Ibid., 40.

34 Ibid., 87.

35 Ibid., 124.

36 Ibid., 125; relevant aspects of the physiology of sound and vibration perception are discussed in chapter 4, 233–4.

37 Ibid., 155.

38 The absence of this set is apparent also in the more recent German edition; *Ludwig Van Beethovens Konversatione Hefte.*

39 Schindler, *Beethoven As I Knew Him*, 230–3.

40 Prod'homme, *Cahiers de conversation*, 216.

41 Ibid., 250.

42 Ibid., 261.

43 Ibid., 275.

44 Ibid., 348.

45 Ibid., 354.

46 Michaux, *Le cas Beethoven*, 203–8; Bankl and Jesserer, *Die Krankheiten Ludwig van Beethovens*, 58.

47 I have not included Franz Wegeler and Gerhard von Breuning in this list. Although both these individuals were physicians, neither was actively involved in his treatment. Beethoven had left Bonn by the time that Wegeler became a physician, and Beethoven died when Breuning was thirteen years old.

48 Schindler, *Beethoven As I Knew Him*, 457.

49 Von Breuning, *Memories of Beethoven*, 7–8.

50 Broman, *The Transformation of German Academic Medicine*, 61.

51 Anderson, Beethoven *Letters*, 1: 57–62.

52 Ibid., 1: 66–8.

53 Ibid., 3: 1412 (my translation).

54 Johann Schmidt, quoted in Thayer, *Ludwig van Beethovens Leben*, 3: 33.

55 Anderson, Beethoven *Letters*, 1: 171–2.

56 Ibid., 1: 66–8.

57 Marek, *Beethoven*, 312.

58 Thayer, *Thayer's Life of Beethoven*, 582–3 and 648.

59 Newman, *The Unconscious Beethoven*, 47–52; for an account of Beethoven's alleged syphilis, see chap. 4, 169–71.

60 Thayer, *Thayer's Life of Beethoven*, 460.

61 Ibid., 1031–2.

62 Anderson, Beethoven *Letters*, 3: 1343.

63 Ibid., 1: 387.

64 Ibid., 2: 685–6.

65 Ibid., 2: 712.

66 Ibid., 2: 818–19.

67 Ibid., 2: 926.

68 Ibid., 2: 946–7.

69 Ibid., 2: 964.

70 Ibid., 2: 971–2.

71 Thayer, *Thayer's Life of Beethoven*, 944.

72 Schindler, *Beethoven As I Knew Him*, 237.

73 Anderson, Beethoven *Letters*, 3: 1037–8.

74 Ibid., 3: 1204.

75 Ibid., 3: 1293.

76 Thayer, *Thayer's Life of Beethoven*, 945–6.

77 Anderson, Beethoven *Letters*, 3: 1038–9.

78 Ibid., 3: 1040.

79 Prod'homme, *Cahiers de Conversation*, 346.

80 Ibid., 348.

81 Ibid., 354.

82 Anderson, Beethoven *Letters*, 3: 1277. There is one further letter from Beethoven to Dr Braunhofer (Anderson, Beethoven *Letters*, 3: 1278); the autograph gives only February as the month of this letter, without providing a specific date. Because of the content of the letters, it is likely that 3: 1278 was written before 3: 1277.

83 Schindler, *Beethoven As I Knew Him*, 318.

84 Nettl, *The Beethoven Encyclopedia*, 40–3. For the complete text of this report, see Appendix 4.

85 Schindler, *Beethoven As I Knew Him*, 457; von Breuning, *Memories of Beethoven*, 89.

86 Schindler, *Beethoven As I Knew Him*, 304.

87 Thayer, *Thayer's Life of Beethoven*, 1059; Michaux, *Le cas Beethoven*, 158; Rolland, *Beethoven the Creator*, 288–90; John Patrick Horan, in Davies, *Beethoven in Person*, 101–3.

88 Thayer, *Thayer's Life of Beethoven*, 1059; for example, Thayer's sentence – "In front of its orifice and towards the tonsils some dimpled scars were observable" – is not in the original Latin.

89 The assistance of Father Frank Morrisey, OMI, of St Paul University, Ottawa, in translating the autopsy report is gratefully acknowledged.

90 Martin, *Beethoven's Hair*.

91 Some of the results of this analysis are available online at http://www.anl.gov/OPA/whatsnew/beethovenstory.htm.

CHAPTER FOUR

1 Marek, *Beethoven*, 326.

2 Ober, "Beethoven"; Edward Larkin, in Cooper, *Beethoven*; Bankl and Jesserer, *Die Krankheiten Ludwig van Beethovens*; Kubba and Young, "Beethoven"; Michaux, *Le cas Beethoven*; Davies, *Beethoven in Person*, 207–14; Keynes, "The Personality, Deafness, and Bad Health of Ludwig van Beethoven."

3 Podolsky and Isselbacher, "Cirrhosis and Alcoholic Liver Disease."

4 Ober, "Beethoven"; Larkin, quoted in Cooper, *Beethoven*; Keynes, "Personality, Deafness, and Bad Health of Beethoven."

5 Podolsky and Isselbacher, "Cirrhosis and Alcoholic Liver Disease."

6 Kubba and Young, "Beethoven"; O'Shea, *Music and Medicine*, 39–65; Davies, *Beethoven in Person*, 85–6.

7 Bankl and Jesserer, *Die Krankheiten Ludwig van Beethovens*, 124–31.

8 Schindler, *Beethoven As I Knew Him*, 47.

9 Ibid., 35.

10 Ibid., 227.

11 Ibid., 164.

12 Ibid., 349n201.

13 Ibid., 357n252.

14 Ibid., 304.

15 Ibid., 385–6.

16 Ibid., 387.

17 Ibid., 458.

18 Prod'homme, *Cahiers de conversation*, 234.

19 Schindler, *Beethoven As I Knew Him*, 304.

20 Ibid., 355n237.

21 Wegeler and Ries, *Beethoven Remembered*, 151.

22 Von Breuning, *Memories of Beethoven*, 89 and 92.

23 Larkin, quoted in Cooper, *Beethoven*, 439–66.

24 Ober, "Beethoven."

25 Thayer, *Thayer's Life of Beethoven*, 943–4.

26 Anderson, Beethoven *Letters*, 1: 111.

27 Johann Schmidt, quoted in Thayer, *Ludwig van Beethovens Leben*, 3: 33

28 Anderson, Beethoven *Letters*, 1: 312–3.

29 Thayer, *Thayer's Life of Beethoven*, 958 and 965.

30 Nettl, *The Beethoven Encyclopedia*, 235–6.

31 Prod'homme, *Cahiers de conversation*, 100–1.

32 Ibid., 152. An amusing incident not directly relevant to Beethoven's over-use of alcohol occurred in November 1822, when Beethoven and a group of friends in a restaurant were in a jocular mood. During the meal, Beethoven must have had one of his serendipitous ideas, and began writing down music in his sketchbook. One of his friends saw this and wrote him a note stating, "You can't stay here till 1922 [100 years later] … you must stop writing music, otherwise the wine will turn sour." Prod'homme, *Cahiers de conversation*, 203–8.

33 Gelder, Mayou, and Geddes, *Psychiatry*, 259–70.

34 Davies, *The Character of a Genius*, 97–104.

35 Martin, *Beethoven's Hair*, 234–8.

36 Goyer, "Trace Elements: Lead"; Taylor, "Usefulness of Measurements of Trace Elements in Hair."

37 Merat, *Traité de la colique métallique*, 111–27 (my translation).

38 Ibid., 99–100.

39 Ibid., 21.

40 Ibid., 26.

41 Ibid., 95.

42 Tourtelle, *Elemens d'hygiène*, 2: 241 (my translation).

43 Ibid., 2: 233–4.

44 Johnson, *Vintage*, 289.

45 Phillips, *A Short History of Wine*, 195.

46 Hunter, *The Diseases of Occupations*, 248–305.

47 Anderson, Beethoven *Letters*, 2: 946–7.

48 Prod'homme, *Cahiers de conversation*, 346.

49 Davies, *Beethoven in Person*, 207–14; Davies, "Beethoven's Nephropathy and Death."

50 Kubba and Young, "Beethoven."

51 Fauci, et al. *Harrison's Principles of Internal Medicine*, 823.

52 Eknoyan, *Primer on Kidney Diseases*, 345–7 and 188–93.

53 Martin, *Beethoven's Hair*, 216–17.

54 Anderson, Beethoven *Letters*, 1: 57–62.

55 Wegeler and Ries, *Beethoven Remembered*, 36.

56 Anderson, Beethoven *Letters*, 3: 1195–6.

57 Ibid., 3: 1095.

58 Thompson, *The Irritable Gut*, 65–84; Heaton and Thompson, *Irritable Bowel Syndrome*.

59 Nettl, *Beethoven Encyclopedia*, 40.

60 Bankl and Jesserer, *Die Krankheiten Ludwig van Beethovens*; Davies, *Beethoven in Person*, 207–14.

61 Merat, *Traité de la colique métallique*, 73.

62 Kubba and Young, "Beethoven"; Davies, *Beethoven in Person*, 174; Davies, "Beethoven's Deafness."

63 Solomon, *Beethoven*, 121–5.

64 Von Breuning, *Memories of Beethoven*, 72.

65 Ealy, "Of Ear Trumpets and a Resonance Plate."

66 Lucente and Har-El, *Essentials of Otolaryngology*, 63.

67 Wegeler and Ries, *Beethoven Remembered*, 108.

68 Prod'homme, *Cahiers de conversation*, 156–7.

69 Anderson, Beethoven *Letters*, 2: 726.

70 Kubba and Young, "Beethoven: A Medical Biography"; Bankl and Jesserer, *Die Krankheiten Ludwig van Beethovens*, 124–31; Kerman and Tyson, *The New Grove Beethoven*, 29–30.

71 Rolland, *Le chant de la resurrection*, 221–7.

72 Solomon, *Beethoven*, 123–4.

73 Keynes, "Personality, Deafness, and Bad Health of Beethoven."

74 Davies, *Beethoven in Person*, 137.

75 Thayer, *Thayer's Life of Beethoven*, 252–3.

76 Kubba and Young, "Beethoven: A Medical Biography"; Davies, *Beethoven in Person*, 174; Davies, "Beethoven's Deafness."

77 Anderson, Beethoven *Letters*, 1: 270–1 and 2: 701.

78 For sources of the dates given in this paragraph, see Table 3.3 in chapter 3, p. 107–8.

79 American Psychiatric Association, *Diagnostic and Statistical Manual of Mental Disorders* (DSMIV), 4th ed. (Washington, DC, 1994).

80 Von Breuning, *Memories of Beethoven*, 44.

81 Wegeler and Ries, *Beethoven Remembered*, 76.

82 Schindler, *Beethoven As I Knew Him*, 226–7.

83 Anderson, Beethoven *Letters*, 21–2.

84 Ibid., 1: 29–30, 122–3, 211–13; Wegeler and Ries, *Beethoven Remembered*, 109.

85 Anderson, Beethoven *Letters*, 3: 1230–1 and 1236–7.

86 American Psychiatric Association, *Diagnostic and Statistical Manual of Mental Disorders,* 629–34.

87 Ibid., 327.

88 Ibid., 338.

89 Anderson, Beethoven *Letters,* 593–4.

90 Ibid., 84; the "Schwan" was a local tavern.

91 Ibid., 1: 32, 35 (letters 33 and 34), and 73–4.

92 Ibid., 1: 268–9.

93 Henderson and Gillespie, *A Text-book of Psychiatry for Students and Practioners,* 124.

94 Davies, *Character of a Genius,* 255–68.

95 Anderson, Beethoven *Letters,* 785.

96 Nettl, *Beethoven Encyclopedia,* 237.

97 Davies, *Beethoven in Person,* 191.

98 Vaughan, Asbury, and Riordan-Eva, *General Ophthalmology,* 30.

99 Ober, "Beethoven: A Medical View."

100 Johann Schmidt, quoted in Thayer, *Ludwig van Beethovens Leben,* 3: 33; Prod'homme, *Cahiers de conversation,* 379.

101 Anderson, Beethoven *Letters,* 3: 1195–6; Prod'homme, *Cahiers de conversation,* 379.

102 Pinel, *Nosographie philosophique,* 2: 529–49.

103 Ibid., 2: 550–69.

104 Michaux, *Le cas Beethoven.*

105 Scheidt, "Quecksilbervergiftung bei Mozart, Beethoven and Schubert."

106 Palferman, "Beethoven"; Drake, "Deafness due to Sarcoid in Ludwig Van Beethoven."

107 Larkin, quoted in Cooper, *Beethoven,* 439–66; Keynes, "Personality, Deafness, and Bad Health of Beethoven."

108 Sharma, "Beethoven's Illness."

109 Jamieson and Wyatt, "Vincent van Gogh's Illness."

110 Grove, *Dictionary of Music and Musicians,* 1: 173.

111 Thayer, *Thayer's Life of Beethoven,* 647–8.

112 Newman, *The Unconscious Beethoven,* 45–52.

113 Kubba and Young, "Beethoven: A Medical Biography"; C. Carpenter, in Scherman and Biancollin, *The Beethoven Companion,*; Palferman, "Beethoven," 112–14; Davies, *Beethoven in Person,* 121–34.

114 Hayden, *Pox,* 71–88.

115 Solomon, *Beethoven*, 262–3. Solomon bases his conclusion that Beethoven frequented prostitutes on correspondence from Beethoven to his bachelor friend, Nikolaus von Zmeskall. Solomon considers that Beethoven used the code word "fortresses" to refer to prostitutes. The following are two (of about five) examples from his letters to Zmeskall. "Be zealous in defending the fortresses of the empire, which, as you know, lost their virginity a long time ago and have already received several assaults," and "Keep away from rotten fortresses, for an attack from them is more deadly than one from well-preserved ones." Solomon concludes from this correspondence that Zmeskall was providing Beethoven with prostitutes. Even if "fortresses" was their code word for prostitutes, it is not clear, after a careful reading of the context of these letters that this indicated that Beethoven was using prostitutes provided to him by Zmeskall.

116 Davies, *Beethoven in Person*, 121–34; Cooper, Letter to the editor.

CHAPTER FIVE

1 Schindler, *Beethoven As I Knew Him*, 324.
2 Grout and Palisca, *A History of Western Music*, 73–7.
3 Cooper, *Beethoven and the Creative Process*.
4 Ibid., 22.
5 Albert and Runco, "A History of Research on Creativity."
6 Richards, "Creativity and Bipolar Mood Swings."
7 Mayer, "Fifty Years of Creativity Research."
8 Gruber, "Aspects of Scientific Discovery."
9 Hayes, "Cognitive Processes in Creativity."
10 Eureka! is the cry allegedly uttered by Archimedes (287–212 BC) when he discovered, while sitting in his bath, the principles governing the upthrust of water that occurred with floating and sinking objects.
11 Sarie Mai, personal communication, 2004, with authorization by Arthur Lackey.
12 Anderson, Beethoven *Letters*, 2: 922–4.
13 Weisberg and O'Hara, "Creativity and Intelligence."
14 Cox, *The Early Mental Traits of Three Hundred Geniuses*.
15 Policastro and Gardner, "From Case Studies to Robust Generalizations."
16 Storr, *The Dynamics of Creation*, 234–51.
17 Rothenberg and Wyshak, "Family Background and Genius."

18 Eisenstadt, "Parental Loss and Genius."

19 Albert, "Family Positions and the Attainment of Eminence."

20 Gaynor and Runco, "Family Size, Birth Order, Age Interval, and the Creativity of Children."

21 Schubert, Wagner, and Schubert, "Family Constellation and Creativity."

22 Howe, "Prodigies and Creativity."

23 Anderson, Beethoven *Letters*, 2: 766–7.

24 Ibid., 2: 797–805.

25 Ibid., 3: 1086–7.

26 Marek, *Beethoven*, 325–7.

27 Prod'homme, *Cahiers de conversation*, 228.

28 Anderson, Beethoven *Letters*, 3: 1141.

29 Prod'homme, *Cahiers de conversation*, 348.

30 L. Schlosser, in Sonneck, *Beethoven*, 132–48. Barry Cooper states that Solomon has concluded that this quotation by Schlosser is almost certainly an invention; *Beethoven and the Creative Process*, 6–7. It is unlikely that Schlosser was quoting Beethoven verbatim. Nevertheless, the broad outlines of the quotation have a ring of truth about Beethoven's compositional method.

31 Schindler, *Beethoven As I Knew Him*, 229.

32 Zatore, "Music and the Brain."

33 Peretz, "Brain Specialization for Music."

34 Brust, "Music and the Neurologist."

35 Hoppe, "Affect, Hemispheric Specialization and Creativity"; van Lancker, "Rags to Riches"; Carlsson and Risberg, "Differences in Frontal Activity between High and Low Creativity Subjects."

36 Restak, "The Creative Brain"; Martindale, "The Biological Basis of Creativity"; Koelsch, et al. "Adults and Children Processing Music."

37 Blakemore, *The Mind Machine*; Becker, *The Mad Genius Controversy*, 23.

38 Terman and Oden, *The Gifted Child Grows Up*.

39 Troyat, *Zola*, 314–15.

40 Becker, *The Mad Genius Controversy*, 61.

41 Slater and Meyer, "Contribution to a Pathography of the Musicians."

42 Hayden, *Pox*, 97–111.

43 McDermott, "Emily Dickinson."

44 Kalian, Lerner, Wiztum, "Creativity and Affective Illness."

45 Prentky, *Creativity and Psychopathology*.

46 Ibid., 54.

47 Ibid., 62.

48 Hans J. Eysenck, *Genius.*

49 Ibid., 8.

50 Simonton, "Creative Productivity, Age and Stress."

51 Andreason, "Creativity and Mental Illness."

52 Post, "Creativity and Psychopathology."

53 Wills, "Forty Lives in the Bepop Business."

54 Ludwig, "Creative Achievement and Psychopathology."

55 Schildkraut, Hirshfield, and Murphy, "Mind and Mood in Modern Art, II."

56 Whybrow, "Of the Muse and Moods Mundane."

57 Schou, "Artistic Productivity and Lithium Prophylaxis in Manic Depressive Illness."

58 Jamison, *Touched with Fire.*

59 Ibid., 49.

60 Ibid., 249.

61 Ibid., 267–70. Jamison does not include Beethoven in her list. In an endnote (297–8) she cites W.A. Frosch, "Moods, Madness and Musical Creativity, I: Major Affective Disease and Musical Creativity," *Comprehensive Psychiatry* 28 (1987): 315–22, who states that Beethoven was "moody" but not "manic-depressive." Jamison appears to concur with this view, although she adds that the possibility Beethoven suffered from a mood disorder cannot be dismissed. Frosch provides no evidence from Beethoven's life, behaviour, or writings to support his conclusion, nor does he review the findings in the context of modern diagnostic criteria.

62 Jamison, *Touched with Fire*, 75.

63 Bower, "Beethoven's Creative Illness."

64 Ellenberger, *The Discovery of the Unconscious*, 888–93.

65 Bower, "Beethoven's Creative Illness," note 69, gives examples from Beethoven's correspondence of what he calls psychotic thinking expressed in letters between 1815 and 1820. It is clear from table 3.3 that Beethoven's psychiatric symptoms were not confined to this period.

66 Prentky, *Creativity and Psychopathology.*

67 MacGregor, *The Discovery of the Art of the Insane*, 25–45.

68 Caldwell, "La Malincola, Final Movement of Beethoven's Quartet, op. 18, no. 6."

69 Solomon, *Mozart*, 491–4.

70 Sweetman, *Van Gogh.*

71 Swafford, *Johannes Brahms*, 614.

72 Waddell, "Creativity and Mental Illness."

73 Rothenberg, *Creativity and Madness*, 115.

74 Holden, *Tchaikovsky*, 316.

75 Whiting, *Satie*, 187.

76 Schildkraut, Hirshfield, and Murphy, "Mind and Mood in Modern Art, II."

77 Post, "Creativity and Psychopathology."

78 Andreason, "Creativity and Mental Illness."

79 Emerson, *The Life of Mussorgsky*, 144.

80 Hanson and Hanson, *The Tragic Life of Toulouse-Lautrec*, 84.

81 Holden, *Tchaikovsky*, 316.

82 Davenport-Hines, *Auden*, 306.

83 Quoted in Trethowan, *Music and Mental Disorder in Music and the Brain*, 399.

84 Holmes, *Coleridge*, 11.

85 Lang, Verret, and Watt, "Drinking and Creativity."

86 Meyers, *Orwell*, 276.

87 Siepmann, *Chopin*, 222.

88 Opitz, "Mozart's Sickness unto Death." Opitz, a physician, cites evidence that Mozart was treated with blood letting during his final illness. As is evident from a review of this topic in chapter 1, blood letting was an accepted treatment for fever during the eighteenth century. In this event, it is probable that "therapeutic" bleeding would have accelerated, and even been the immediate cause of his death. This could also explain the precipitate and furtive circumstances of his funeral and burial.

89 Solomon, *Mozart: A Life*, 491–4.

90 Honan, *Jane Austen*, 385.

91 Simonton, "The Swan-song Phenomenon."

92 Post, "Creativity and Psychopathology."

93 Hood, "Deafness in Musicians."

94 Ibid., 336.

95 Ibid., 338.

96 Ibid., 343.

97 Solomon, *Beethoven*, 121–5.

BIBLIOGRAPHY

Albert, Robert. "Family Positions and the Attainment of Eminence: A Study of Special Family Position and Special Family Experiences." *Gifted Child Quarterly* 24 (1980): 87–95.

Albert, Robert, and Mark Runco. "A History of Research on Creativity." In *Handbook of Creativity*, ed. Richard J. Sternberg. New York: Cambridge University Press, 1999.

Albrecht, Theodore. *Letters to Beethoven and Other Correspondence.* 3 vols. Lincoln, NE: University of Nebraska Press, 1996.

Alterman, K. "Diagnostic Challenge: Recurrent Infections, Diarrhea, Ascites, and Phonophobia in a 57 year old man." *Canadian Medical Association* 15 (1982): 623–8.

American Psychiatric Association. *Diagnostic and Statistical Manual of Mental Disorders* (DSM-IV) 4th ed. Washington, DC, 1994.

Anderson, Emily. *The Letters of Beethoven.* 3 vols. New York: St Martin's Press, 1961.

Andreason, Nancy. "Creativity and Mental Illness." *American Journal of Psychiatry* 144 (1987): 1288–92.

Baillie, Matthew. *The Morbid Anatomy in Some of the Most Important Parts of the Human Body.* London: W. Bulmer, 1793.

Bankl, Hans, and Hans Jesserer. *Die Krankheiten Ludwig van Beethovens: Pathographie seines Lebens und Pathologic seiner Leiden.* Wien: Verlag Wilhelm Maudrich, 1987.

Beaumont, William. *The Physiology of Digestion*. 2nd ed. Burlington, VT: Chauncey Goodrich, 1847.

Becker, G. *The Mad Genius Controversy: A Study in the Sociology of Deviance*. Beverly Hills, CA: Sage, 1978.

Beethoven, Ludwig van. *Ludwig Van Beethovens Konversatione Hefte*. 9 vols. Leipzig: Deutscher Verlag für Musik, 1976.

BIS CD – 406/407.

Blakemore, C. *The Mind Machine*. London: BBC Books, 1988.

Bower, H. "Beethoven's Creative Illness." *Australia and New Zealand Journal of Psychiatry* 23 (1989): 111–16.

Brandenburg, Sieghard. *Briefwechsel Gesamtausgabe*. 7 vols. Munich: Henle, 1996–1998.

Braudel, Ferdinand. *The Structures of Everyday Life*. Trans. Sian Reynolds. 3 vols. New York: Harper and Row, 1981.

Broman, Thomas. *The Transformation of German Academic Medicine. 1750–1820*. Cambridge University Press 1996.

Brust, John. "Music and the Neurologist." *Annals of the New York Academy of Sciences* 930 (2001): 143–52.

Buch, Esteban. *Beethoven's Ninth: A Political History*. Trans. Richard Miller. Chicago, University of Chicago Press, 2003. First published in French as *La neuvième de Beethoven: une histoire politique*. Paris: Gallimard, 1999.

Caldwell, A. "La Malincola: Final Movement of Beethoven's Quartet op 18, no. 6 – Musical Account of Manic Depressive States." *Journal of the American Medical Women's Association* 27 (1972): 241–8.

Carlsson, I., P.E. Wendt, and J. Risberg. "Differences in Frontal Activity between High and Low Creativity Subjects." *Neuropsychologia* 38 (2000): 873–85.

Carpenter, Charles. *The Beethoven Companion*. Ed. Thomas Scherman and Louis Biancolli. Garden City, New York: Doubleday 1972.

Chapman, Nathaniel. *Elements of Therapeutics and Materia Medica*. 4th ed., 2 vols. Philadelphia: H.C. Carey, 1825.

Closson, E. *L'élément flamand dans Beethoven*. Bruxelles: Imprimerie Veuve Monnom, 1928.

Coley, N. "Physicians, Chemists and the Analysis of Mineral Waters: The Most Difficult Part of Chemistry." In *The Medical History of Spas*, ed. Roy Porter, 56–66, London: Wellcome Institute of Medicine, 1990.

Cooper, Barry. *Beethoven*. New York: Oxford University Press, 2000.

– *Beethoven and the Creative Process*. Oxford: Clarendon Press, 1990.

– Letter to the Editor. *Beethoven Journal* 14 (1999): 102.

Cooper, Martin, ed. *Beethoven: The Last Decade*. New York: Oxford University Press, 1985.

Cox, C.M. "The Early Mental Traits of 300 Geniuses." In *Genetic Studies of Genius*, ed. L.M. Terman. Stanford, CA: Stanford University Press, 1926.

Davenport-Hines, R. *Auden*. London: Heinemann, 1995.

Davies, Norman. *Europe: A History*. Oxford: Oxford University Press, 1995.

Davies, Peter. *Beethoven in Person: His Deafness, Illnesses and Death*, Westport, CT: Greenwood Press, 2001.

– "Beethoven's Deafness: A New Theory." *Medical Journal of Australia* 149 (1988): 644–9.

– "Beethoven's Nephropathy and Death: Discussion Paper." *Journal of the Royal Society of Medicine* 86 (1993): 159–61.

– *The Character of Genius: Beethoven in Perspective*. Westport, CT: Greenwood Press, 2002.

De Nora, Tia. *Beethoven and the Construction of Genius: Musical Politics in Vienna, 1792–1803*. Los Angeles: University of California Press, 1995.

Didier, Beatrice. *La musique des lumières*. Paris: Presses universitaires de France, 1985.

Donnenberg, M., M. Collins, et al. "The Sound That Failed." *American Journal of Medicine* 108 (2000): 475–80.

Drake, E. "Deafness Due to Sarcoid in Ludwig van Beethoven." *Neurology* 44 (1994): 564.

Durant, Will and Ariel. *The Age of Voltaire: A History of Civilization in Western Europe from 1715–1756, The Story of Civilization*, vol. 9. New York: Simon and Schuster, 1965.

– *Rousseau and Revolution: A History of Civilization in France, England, and Germany from 1756, and in the Remainder of Europe from 1715 to 1789, The Story of Civilization*, vol. 10. New York: Simon and Schuster, 1967.

Ealy, George Thomas. "Of Ear Trumpets and Resonance Plates: Early Hearing Aids and Beethoven's Hearing Perception." *Nineteenth Century Music* 17, 3 (1993–94): 262–73.

Eisenstadt, J. "Parental Loss and Genius." *American Journal of Psychology* 33 (1978): 211–23.

Eknoyan, G. *A Primer on Kidney Diseases*. San Diego, CA: Academic Press, 1998.

Ellenberger, Henri. *The Discovery of the Unconscious*. New York: Basic Books, 1970.

Emerson, C. *The Life of Mussorgsky*. London: Cambridge University Press, 1999.

Eysenck, Hans. *Genius: The Natural History of Creativity*. London: Cambridge University Press, 1995.

Fauci, A., et al. *Harrison's Principles of Internal Medicine*, 14th ed. New York: McGraw-Hill, 1998.

Fischer-Homberger. "E. Germany and Austria." In *World History of Psychiatry*, ed. John Howells, 256–90. London: Baillière Tindall, 1975.

Frank, Johann. *System einer vollständigen medizenischen Polizey*. Vienna: 1817.

Furbank, P. *Diderot*. London: Minerva, 1992.

Gaynor, J., and M. Rumco. "Family Size, Birth Order, Age Interval, and the Creativity of Children." *Journal of Creative Behaviour* 26 (1992): 108–17.

Gelder, M., R. Mayou, and J. Geddes. *Psychiatry*. 2nd ed. Oxford University Press, 1999.

Goyer, R. "Trace Elements: Lead." In *Handbook of Clinical Chemistry*, ed. Mario Werner, 4: 229–41. Boca Raton: CPC Press, 1989.

Grout, Donald, and Claude Palisca. *A History of Western Music*. 5th ed. New York: Norton, 1996.

Grove, George, ed. *A Dictionary of Music and Musicians*. 4 vols. London: Mac-Millan, 1879.

Gruber, H. "Aspects of Scientific Discovery: Aesthetics and Cognition." In *Creativity*, ed. John Brockman, 48–74. New York: Simon and Schuster, 1993.

Hanson, Lawrence, and Elisabeth Hanson. *The Tragic Life of Toulouse-Lautrec*. London: Secker and Warburg, 1956.

Hayden, Deborah. *Pox: Genius, Madness, and the Mysteries of Syphilis*. New York: Basic Books, 2003.

Hayes, J. "Cognitive Processes in Creativity." In *Handbook of Creativity*, ed. J. Glover, R. Ronning, and C. Reynolds, 135–45. New York: Plenum Press, 1989.

Heaton, K., and W. Grant Thompson. *Irritable Bowel Syndrome*. Oxford: Health Press, 1999.

Henderson, D., and R. Gillespie. *A Text-book of Psychiatry for Students and Practioners*. Oxford University Press, 1927.

Herriot, Edouard. *La Vie de Beethoven*, Paris: Galimard, 1928.

Holden, A. *Tchaikovsky*. New York: Viking Press, 1995.

Holmes, R. *Coleridge*. New York: Pantheon, 1998.

Honan, P. *Jane Austen: Her Life*. London: Weidenfeld and Nicholson, 1987.

Hood, D. "Deafness in Musicians." In *Music and the Brain*, ed. M. Critchley and R. Henson, 323–43. Springfield, IL: CC Thomas, 1997.

Hoppe, K. "Affect, Hemispheric Specialization and Creativity." In *Creativity and Affect*, ed. M. Shaw and M. Runco, 213–24. Norwood, NJ: Abex, 1994.

Howe, Michael, "Prodigies and Creativity." In *Handbook of Creativity*, ed. Robert J. Sternberg, 431–46. New York: Cambridge University Press, 1999.

Hunter, Donald. *The Diseases of Occupations*. 8th ed. New York: Oxford University Press, 1994.

Jamison, Kay. *Touched with Fire: Manic Depressive Temperament and the Artistic Temperament*. New York: MacMillan Free Press, 1993.

Jamison, K., and R. Wyatt. "Vincent van Gogh's Illness." *British Medical Journal* 304 (1992): 577.

Jeanclaude, Georgette. *Un amour de Beethoven: Marie Bigot de Morogues*. Strasbourg: Oberlin, 1992.

Jenner, Edward. *An Inquiry into the Causes and Effects of Cow Pox*. London: Sampson Low, 1798.

Johnson, H. *Vintage: The Story of Wine*. New York: Simon and Schuster, 1989.

Jordanova, L. "Reflections on Medical Reform: Cabanis' Coup d'oeil." In *Medicine in the Enlightenment*, ed. Roy Porter, 166–80. Amsterdam: Rodopi, 1995.

Kalian, M., V. Lerner, and E. Wiztum. "Creativity and Affective Illness." *American Journal of Psychiatry* 159 (2002): 675–6.

Kerman, Joseph, and Alan Tyson. *The New Grove Beethoven*. New York: Norton, 1983.

Keynes, M. "The Personality, Deafness, and Bad Health of Ludwig van Beethoven." *Journal of Medical Biography* 10 (2002): 46–57.

Kinderman, William. *Beethoven*. Oxford: Oxford University Press, 1995.

Knight, Frida. *Beethoven and the Age of Revolution*. London: Camelot, 1973.

Koelsch, Stephan, et al. "Adults and Children Processing Music: An fMRI Study." *NeuroImage*, 25 (2005): 1068–76.

Krieger, Leonard. *Kings and Philosophers: 1689–1789*. New York: Norton, 1970.

Krizek, V. "History of Balneotherapy." In *Medical Hydrology*, ed. Sidney Licht, 131–59. Baltimore, MD: Waverly, 1963.

Kubba, A., and M. Young. "Beethoven: A Medical Biography." *Lancet* 347 (1996): 167–75.

Küster, Konrad. *Mozart: A Musical Biography*. Oxford: Clarendon, 1996.

Lande, Lawrence. *Beethoven and Quebec*. Foundations for Canadian Historical Research Publications 2, Montreal, Redpath Library, McGill University, 1966.

Lang, A., L. Verret, and C. Watt. "Drinking and Creativity: Objective and Subjective Effects." *Addictive Behaviour* 9 (1984): 395–9.

Libby, Denis. "Italy: Two Opera Centres." In *Man and Music: The Classical Era*, ed. Neal Zaslow, 15–60. London: MacMillan, 1989.

Lindemann, Mary. *Health and Healing in Eighteenth-century Germany*. Baltimore, MD: Johns Hopkins University Press, 1996.

Lockwood, Lewis. *Beethoven: The Music and the Life*. New York: Norton, 2003.

Lucente, F., and G. Har-El. *Essentials of Otolaryngology*. Philadelphia: Lippincott, Williams and Wilkins, 1999.

Ludwig, A. "Creative Achievement and Psychopathology: Comparison Among Professions." *American Journal of Psychotherapy* 46 (1992): 330–56.

Lund, Susan. "Beethoven: A True 'Fleshly Father'?" *Beethoven Newsletter* 3 (1988): 1–11 and 25–40.

MacGregor, John. *The Discovery of the Art of the Insane*. Princeton, NJ: Princeton University Press, 1989.

Maehle, Andreas-Holger. "Conflicting Attitudes towards Inoculation in Enlightenment Germany." In *Medicine in the Enlightenment*, ed. Roy Porter, 198–222. Amsterdam: Rodopi, 1995.

Mai, François. "Beaumont's Contribution to Gastric Psychophysiology: A Reappraisal." *Canadian Journal of Psychiatry* 33 (1988): 650–6.

– "Beethoven's Terminal Illness and Death." *Journal of the Royal College of Physicians of Edinburgh 36* (2006): 258–63.

Marek, George R. *Beethoven: Biography of a Genius*. New York: Funk and Wagnalls, 1969.

Martin, Russell. *Beethoven's Hair*. New York: Broadway, 2000.

Martindale, Colin. "The Biological Basis of Creativity." In *Handbook of Creativity*, ed. Robert Sternberg, 137–52. New York: Cambridge University Press, 1999.

Marx, H. "Beethoven, l'homme politique." In *Ludwig van Beethoven, 1770–1970*. Bonn: Internationes, 1970.

Mayer, Richard. "Fifty Years of Creativity Research." In *Handbook of Creativity*, ed. Robert Sternberg, 449–60. New York: Cambridge University Press, 1999.

McDermott, J. "Emily Dickinson: A Study of Periodicity in Her Work." *American Journal of Psychiatry* 158 (2001): 686–90.

Mellers, Wilfrid, *Beethoven and the Voice of God.* London: Faber and Faber, 1983.

Merat, François. *Traité de la Colique Metallique.* Paris: Melpignon-Marvis, 1812.

Meredith, William. "The History of Beethoven's Skull Fragments," *Beethoven Journal* 20, 1–2 (2005): 3–39.

Meyers, J. *Orwell: Wintry Conscience of a Generation.* New York: Norton, 2000.

Michaux, Jean-Louis, *Le cas Beethoven: le génie et le malade.* Bruxelles: Édition Racine, 1999.

Mongrédien, Jean. "Paris: The End of the Ancien Régime." In *Man and Music: The Classical Era,* ed. Neal Zaslow, 61–98. London: MacMillan, 1989.

Nettl, Paul. *The Beethoven Encyclopedia.* New York: Citadel, 1994.

Newman, Ernest. *The Unconscious Beethoven: An Essay in Musical Psychology,* London: Parsons, 1927.

O'Shea, John. *Music and Medicine: Medical Profiles of Great Composers.* London: Dent, 1990.

Ober, W. "Beethoven: A Medical View." *The Practitioner* 205 (1970): 819–24.

Opitz, John. "Mozart's Sickness unto Death." Prepared for the Symposium: Mozart in Montana – A Humanistic 200 Years Commemoration. Montana State University, 1991.

Palferman, T.G. "Beethoven: A Medical Biography." *Journal of Medical Biography* 1 (1993): 35–45.

Peretz, Isabelle. "Brain Specialization for Music: New Evidence from Congenital Amusia." *Annals of the New York Academy of Sciences* 930 (2001): 153–65.

Pfeiffer, Carl J. *The Art and Practice of Western Medicine in the Early Nineteenth Century.* Jefferson, NC: McFarland, 1985.

Phillips, Rod. *A Short History of Wine.* New York: Penguin, 2000.

Pinel, Phillipe. *Nosographie philosophique ou La méthode de l'analyse appliquée à la médicine.* 6ᵉ ed., 3 vols. Paris: J.A. Brosson, 1818.

Podolsky, D., and K. Isselbacher. "Cirrhosis and Alcoholic Liver Disease." In *Harrison's Principles of Internal Medicine, Companion Handbook,* ed. Anthony Franci et al., 1704–09. 14th ed. New York: McGraw Hill, 1998.

Policastro, Emma, and Howard Gardner. "From Case Studies to Robust Generalizations: An Approach to the Study of Creativity." In *Handbook of Creativity,* ed. Robert J. Sternberg, 213–25. New York: Cambridge University Press, 1999.

Post, Felix. "Creativity and Psychopathology: A Study of 291 World-Famous Men." *British Journal of Psychiatry* 165 (1994): 22–34.

Prentky, R.A. *Creativity and Psychopathology: A Neurocognitive Perspective.* New York: Praeger, 1980.

Prod'homme, Jacques-Gabriel, ed. *Cahiers de conversation de Beethoven.* Paris: Correa, 1946.

Restak, Richard. "The Creative Brain." In *Creativity*, ed. John Brockman, 164–75. New York: Simon and Schuster, 1993.

Rice, John A. "Vienna under Joseph II and Leopold II." In *The Classical Era: From the 1740s to the End of the 18th Century*, ed. Neal Zaslow, 127–57. London: Macmillan, 1989.

Richards, Ruth. "Creativity and Bipolar Mood Swings: Why the Association?" In *Creativity and Affect*, ed. M. Shaw and M. Runco, 44–72. Norwood, NJ: Abex, 1994.

Rolland, Romain. *Beethoven the Creator: From the Appassionata to the Eroica.* Trans. Ernest Newman. Garden City, NY: Garden City Publishing, 1937.

– *Le chant de la resurrection.* Paris: Sablier, 1937.

Rothenberg, A., and G. Wyshak. "Family Background and Genius." *Canadian Journal of Psychiatry* 49 (2004): 185–91.

Rothenberg, A. *Creativity and Madness.* Baltimore: MD: Johns Hopkins University Press, 1990.

Rousseau, Jean-Jacques. "Léttre sur la musique française." In *Source Readings in Music History: The Classic Era*, ed. Oliver Strunk, 62–80. New York: Norton, 1965.

Scheidt, W. "Quecksilbervergiftung bei Mozart, Beethoven and Schubert." *Medizinishe Klinik* 62 (1967): 195.

Scheminsky, F. "Austria." In *Medical Hydrology*, ed. Sidney Licht, 488–95. Baltimore, MD: Waverley, 1963.

Schildkraut, J., A. Hirshfield, and J. Murphy. "Mind and Mood in Modern Art, II: Depressive Disorders, Spirituality, and Early Deaths in the Abstract Expressionist Artists of the New York School." *American Journal of Psychiatry* 151 (1994): 482–8.

Schindler, Anton. *Beethoven As I Knew Him.* Ed. Donald MacArdle, trans. Constance Jolly. New York: Dover, 1996.

Schlosser, Johann Aloys. *Beethoven: The First Biography, 1827.* Ed. Barry Cooper, trans. Reinhard G. Pauly. Portland, OR: Amadeus, 1995.

Schmidt-Görg, Joseph. *Ludwig Van Beethoven. 1770–1970.* Bonn: Inter-Nationes, 1970.

Schou, Mogens. "Artistic Productivity and Lithium Prophylaxis in Manic Depressive Illness." *British Journal of Psychiatry* 135 (1979): 97–103.

Schubert, D., M. Wagner, and H. Schubert. "Family Constellation and Creativity: First-born Predominance among Classical Music Composers." *Journal of Clinical Psychology* 95 (1977): 147–9.

Shackleton, Robert. "The Enlightenment: Free Inquiry and the World of Ideas." In *The Eighteenth Century: Europe in the Age of Enlightenment*, ed. Alfred Cobban, 260–78. New York: McGraw-Hill, 1969.

Sharma, O. "Beethoven's Illness: Whipple's Disease rather than Sarcoidosis?" *Journal of the Royal Society Medicine* 87 (1994): 383–5.

Shedlock, J.S., trans. and ed. *Beethoven's Letters: A Critical Edition with Explanatory Notes.* London: Dent, 1909.

Siepmann, J. *Chopin, The Reluctant Romantic.* Boston: Northeastern University Press, 1995.

Simonton, D. "Creative Productivity, Age and Stress: A Biographical Time-Series Analysis of Ten Classical Composers." *Journal of Personality and Social Psychology* 35 (1977): 791–804.

– "The Swan-song Phenomenon: Last Works Effects for 172 Classical Composers in Genius and Creativity." *Psychology and Aging* 4 (1989): 42–7.

Slater, Eliot, and Adolph Meyer. "Contribution to a Pathography of the Musicians: 1. Robert Schumann." *Confinia Psychiatrica* 2 (1959): 65–94.

Solomon, Maynard. *Beethoven.* London: Cassell, 1978.

– *Mozart: A Life.* New York: Harper Collins, 1995.

Sonneck, Oscar George, ed. *Beethoven: Impressions by His Contemporaries.* New York: Dover, 1967.

Sournia, Jean-Charles. *Illustrated History of Medicine.* London: Harold Starke, 1992.

Spiel, Hilde. *The Congress of Vienna: An Eye-Witness Account.* Trans. Richard H. Weber. Philadelphia: Chilton, 1968.

Sterba, Editha, and Richard Sterba. *Beethoven and His Nephew: A Psychoanalytic Study of their Relationship.* New York: Schocken, 1971.

Storr, Anthony. *The Dynamics of Creation.* Harmondsworth: Penguin, 1976.

Swafford, J. *Johannes Brahms: A Biography.* New York: Alfred Knopf, 1997.

Sweetman, D. *Van Gogh: His Life and His Art.* London: Crown, 1990.

Taylor, A. "Usefulness of Measurements of Trace Elements in Hair." *Annals of Clinical Biochemistry* 23 (1986): 364–78.

Terman, L.M., and M. Oden. *The Gifted Child Grows Up: Twenty-five Years Follow up of a Superior Group*. Vol. 4 of *Genetic Studies of Genius*. Stanford, CA: Stanford University Press, 1947.

Thayer, Alexander Wheelock, *Ludwig van Beethovens Leben: nach dem Original Manuskript deutsch bearbeitet von Hermann Deiters*. 3 vols. New York: G. Olms, Hildascheim, 1971.

– *Thayer's Life of Beethoven*. Rev. and ed. Elliot Forbes. Princeton, NJ: Princeton University Press, 1967.

Thompson, W. Grant. *The Irritable Gut: Functional Disorders of the Alimentary Canal*. Baltimore: University Park Press, 1979.

Thomson, Samuel. *New Guide To Health: or Botanic Family Physician*. 3rd ed. Boston: 1832.

Tourtelle, Étienne. *Élémens d'hygiène ou l'influence des choses physiques et morales sur l'homme, et de moyens de conserver la santé*. 2 vols. Paris: Rémont, 1815.

Tovey, Donald Francis. *Beethoven*. London: Oxford University Press, 1964.

Trethowan, W. "Music and Mental Disorder." In *Music and the Brain*, ed. Macdonald Critchley and R.A. Henson, 398–412. Springfield, IL: C.L. Thomas, 1977.

Troyat, Henri. *Zola*. Paris: Flammarion, 1992.

van Lancker, Diana. "Rags to Riches: Our Increasing Appreciation of Cognitive and Communicative Abilities of the Human Right Cerebral Hemisphere." *Brain and Language* 57 (1997): 1–11.

Vaughan, D., T. Asbury, and P. Riordan-Eva. *General Ophthalmology*. Norwalk, CT: Appleton and Lange, 1995.

Von Breuning, Gerhard. *Memories of Beethoven: From the House of the Black-robed Spaniards*, ed. Maynard Solomon, trans Henry Mins and Maynard Solomon. Cambridge: Cambridge University Press, 1992.

Waddell, C. "Creativity and Mental Illness: Is There a Link?" *Canadian Journal of Psychiatry* 43 (1998): 166–72.

Webster, James. "The Falling-out between Haydn and Beethoven: The Evidence of the Sources." in *Beethoven Essays: Studies in Honor of Elliot Forbes*, ed. Lewis Lockwood and Phyllis Benjamin, 3–45. Cambridge, MA: Harvard University Press, 1984.

Wegeler, Franz, and Ferdinand Ries. *Beethoven Remembered: The Biographical Notes of Franz Wegeler and Ferdinand Ries.* Arlington, VA: Great Ocean, 1987.

Weisberg, Robert W., and Linda O'Hara. "Creativity and Intelligence." In *Handbook of Creativity*, ed. Robert Sternberg, 251–72. New York: Cambridge University Press, 1999.

Whiting, S. *Satie: The Bohemian.* Oxford: Clarendon Press, 1999.

Whybrow, P. "Of the Muse and Moods Mundane." *American Journal of Psychiatry* 151 (1994): 477–9.

Williams, Joseph. *Treatise on the Ear: Including Its Anatomy, Physiology and Pathology.* Edinburgh: John Churchill, 1840.

Wills, Geoffrey. "Forty Lives in the Bepop Business: Mental Health in a Group of Eminent Jazz Musicians." *British Journal Psychiatry* 183 (2003): 255–9.

Withering, William. *An Account of the Foxglove and Some of its Medical Uses.* Birmingham: M. Swinney, 1785.

Zatore, Robert. "Music and the Brain." *Annals of the New York Academy of Sciences* 999 (2003): 4–14.

INDEX